ENCYCLOPEDIA OF GOOD HEALTH

NUTRITION

ENCYCLOPEDIA OF GOOD HEALTH

NUTRITION

Series Editors

MARIO ORLANDI, Ph.D., M.P.H.

and

DONALD PRUE, Ph.D.

Text by

ANNETTE SPENCE

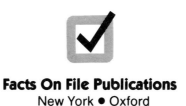

Facts On File Publications
New York • Oxford

A FRIEDMAN GROUP BOOK

First published in 1988 by Facts On File Publications, Inc.
460 Park Avenue South
New York, New York 10016

Library of Congress Cataloging-in-Publication Data

Spence, Annette.
Nutrition.

(Encyclopedia of good health)
Includes index.
Summary: Examines the major food groups, what effect they have on the body, what foods are good nutritional choices, and how good eating habits can be developed.
1. Nutrition—Juvenile literature. 2. Food—Juvenile literature. [1. Nutrition.
2. Food] I. Title. II. Series: Spence, Annette. Encyclopedia of good health.
TX 355.S66   1988   613.2   87-20203
ISBN 0-8160-1670-4

British CIP data available upon request

ENCYCLOPEDIA OF GOOD HEALTH: NUTRITION
was prepared and produced by
Michael Friedman Publishing Group, Inc.
15 West 26th Street
New York, New York 10010

Designer: Rod Gonzalez
Art Director: Mary Moriarty
Illustrations: Kenneth Spengler

Typeset by BPE Graphics, Inc.
Color separated, printed, and bound in Hong Kong by South Seas International Press Company Ltd.

1 3 5 7 9 10 8 6 4 2

About the Series Editors

Mario Orlandi is chief of the Division of Health Promotion Research of the American Health Foundation. He has a Ph.D. in psychology with further study in health promotion. He has written and edited numerous books and articles, among them The American Health Foundation Guide to Lifespan Health *(Dodd Mead, 1984), and has received numerous grants, awards, and commendations. Orlandi lives in New York City.*

Dr. Donald M. Prue is a management consultant specializing in productivity improvement and wellness programs in business and industrial settings. He was formerly a senior scientist at the American Health Foundation and holds a doctorate in clinical psychology. He has published over forty articles and books on health promotion and was recognized in the Congressional Record *for his work. Prue lives in Houston, Texas.*

About the Author

Annette Spence received a degree in journalism from the University of Tennessee at Knoxville. Her articles have appeared in Redbook, Weight Watchers Magazine, Cosmopolitan, *and* Bride's, *and she has contributed to a number of books. Spence is associate editor for Whittle Communications, a health media company in New York City. She lives in Stamford, Connecticut.*

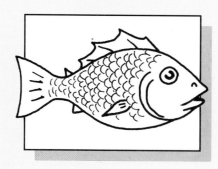

E N T S

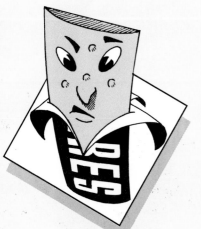

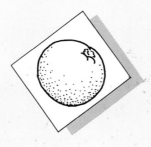

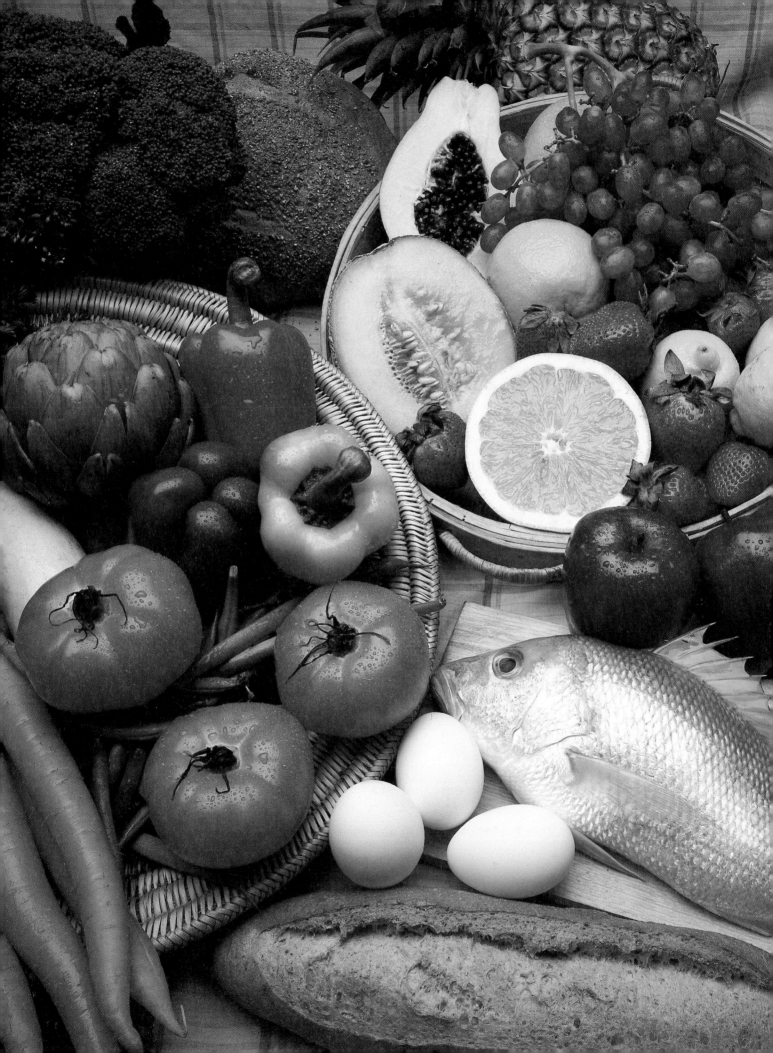

How to Use This Book

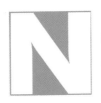

N utrition is part of a six-volume encyclopedia series of books on health topics significant to junior-high students. These health topics are closely related to each other, and for this reason, you'll see references to the other volumes in the series appearing throughout the book. You'll also see references to the other pages *within* this book. These references are important because they tell you where you can find more interrelated and interesting information on the specific subject at hand.

Like each of the books in the series, this book is divided into two sections. The first section tells you why it's a good idea for you to know about this health topic and how it affects you. The second section helps you find ways to improve and maintain your health. We include quizzes and plans designed to help you see how these health issues are relative to you. It's your responsibility to take advantage of them and apply them to your life. Even though this book was written expressly for you and other people your age, you are the one who's in control of learning from it and exercising good health habits for the rest of your life.

What's Important For Me To Know About Nutrition?

Nutrition is more than words and charts in a textbook. It's the doughnut you ate on the bus this morning, the tuna fish casserole that is being served in the school cafeteria, the apple you've stashed in your locker. Nutrition has a lot to do with how you feel today and how healthy you'll be tomorrow. Once you eliminate all the boring stuff and get right down to what *you* need to know, there's nothing hard to understand about nutrition. You'll be surprised to see how simple it really is.

As a teen, you've come a long way, but you've still got a lot of growing to do—which is why your body needs good nutrition on a daily basis.

Nutrition is the key to feeling and looking good.

You missed lunch at school (band practice went over fifteen minutes), and then Mom didn't have dinner ready before it was time to leave for the ball game. You made up for it with a hot dog and soda during the third quarter.

Maybe you're one of those people who can go for days without a real meal. Or maybe you've been known to eat a whole pizza at one sitting. On the other hand, maybe there have been times when you felt a little out of sync—not exactly sick, but not 100 percent healthy, either. The truth is, you're at the age when the cause could be totally hormonal (see ''Human Sexuality'').

At the same time, you're not at the age when three square meals and Recommended Daily Allowances are your big priorities—even if they should be. So it probably won't surprise you to

hear that the hot dog eaten twelve hours after your last meal could be the reason you don't exactly feel great. Nutrition is a fundamental part of what makes your body work—and keep on working.

Energy and Performance

Food is one of the body's basic needs, and when the body doesn't get what it needs—whether you're not eating at all or you're eating foods with little nutritional value (we'll talk about that hot dog later)—the body reacts by slowing down. Maybe you feel fine now, but sooner or later, you'll notice that climbing stairs wears you out. Or you can't concentrate on your algebra. You're tired, and nutrition—or the lack of it—could be the cause.

An adequate diet can make you feel even better than 100 percent. It's been shown that students who eat breakfast do better in school. And any athlete will swear by a diet rich in high-energy complex carbohydrates.

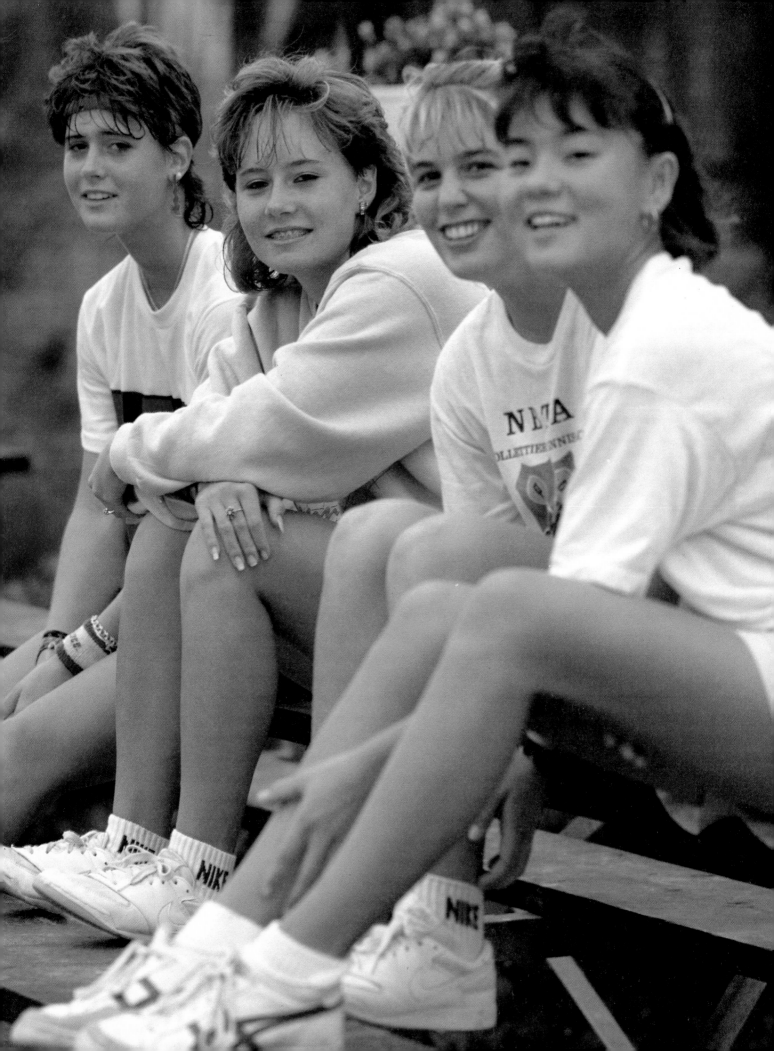

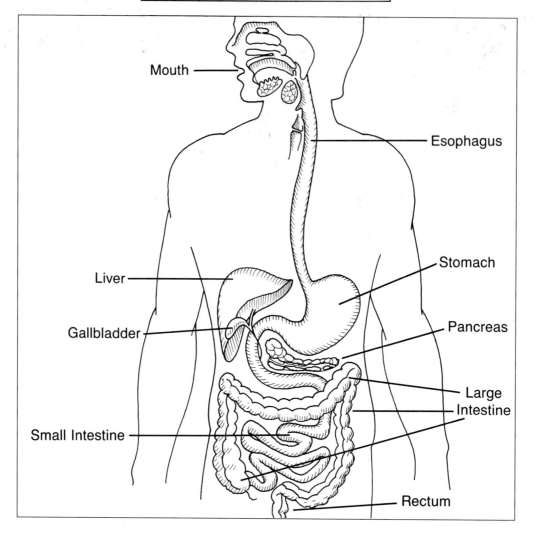

Mouth

Esophagus

Liver

Stomach

Gallbladder

Pancreas

Large Intestine

Small Intestine

Rectum

W *hat* **Really** *Happens* **When** *You* **Eat?**

After that hot dog disappeared into your mouth, it made its way down the esophagus, through the stomach and into the small intestine, where the major part of digestion takes place: Food is broken down into nutrients small enough to be absorbed into the bloodstream. The bloodstream carries the nutrients to all parts of the body, and *that's* where you get the energy to do the things you do every day. Nutrition not only boosts the muscles you use, it also provides energy to keep up the things you don't think about: the building and repairing of cells and the movement of blood through your body.

What Really Happens When You Don't Eat?

In the time between the bowl of cereal you ate this morning to the hot dog you ate during the third quarter, your body was still functioning. Humans aren't like cars; we can keep going for a while, even when no fuel is provided. However, you weren't operating at peak energy because without food, your blood sugar level dropped. The result: You felt tired and irritable. Unfed, your body began to reach out for the next best thing—stored fat *and* the protein in your muscles and organs. This weakens you and could eventually make you sick. Some recent research also shows that you might be increasing your chance of gaining weight. Your body thinks it's starving when you don't eat, so it slows down and saves all the food you ate yesterday and before. By the time you *do* eat, it's stockpiled for the next bout of starvation.

Diseases

You're probably well aware of the research linking nutrition with our most common diseases. Though we've always known that poor nutrition lowers our resistance to illness, lately it's been made startlingly clear just how our eating habits affect our health.

Now, as a teenager, you may not be overly concerned with how your food choices might affect you when you are 45. However, there are diseases you may avoid by making the right decisions now—or helping someone else to.

Chances are good you've known someone who has had *cancer* for it's second only to heart disease as a cause of death in the United States. Scientists have identified more than 300 varieties of cancer, all characterized by an uncontrolled and irregular growth of abnormal cells. Although other risk factors—family history, tobacco and alcohol use, and even stress and exercise—come into play, a healthy diet is at the top—next to stopping smoking—on the risk-reducer list (see "Substance Abuse").

It's been proven more than once that food choices make a big difference in cancer risk. The general rule: A diet heavy in fatty foods (marbled meats, high-fat dairy products, processed or packaged foods) and low in natural, fibrous foods (fruits, vegetables, whole grains) increases cancer risk.

Here's how scientists see the food-cancer connection: When the diet is high in fat and cholesterol, bacteria inside of us break it down into cancer-causing substances. In our world, it's hard to avoid all fatty and cholesterol-heavy foods, so doctors advise us to cut down as much as possible on fat and cholesterol and to load up on fiber-rich foods. Fiber works *against* cancer because it comes from plants, and some plant parts can't be digested. Those parts bulk up your waste and speed it out of the body. With it, the waste takes along those cancerous substances that might have stuck to the colon (the path out of the body). Fiber helps get rid of many of these cancerous substances because it moves them out quicker than usual.

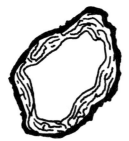
Normal Artery

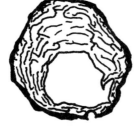
Artery with Fatty Deposits

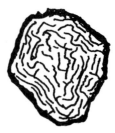
Clogged Artery

The illustration above shows what an artery looks like as it becomes clogged, which will help you understand how a heart attack happens. These arteries are actually like long tubes, and intermittently, sections of them will be coated with more fatty deposits than in other places. The blood coursing through the arteries all of a sudden comes to an area where it can not pass easily. Imagine what happens when there is an accident or a stalled car on a highway—a terrific traffic jam and a lot of aggravated people.

We also know that vitamins A and C help prevent cancer. At the same time, other substances, such as food preservatives (see "Cholesterol, Sodium, and Additives," page 46), have been shown to cause cancer in animals. Do they affect humans? Some do, some we're not sure of. Research to answer these and other questions about cancer is ongoing, which is why it's important to remember that no one vitamin or nutrient has been proven to absolutely prevent cancer. While we're still learning it doesn't hurt to say over and over again: A high-fiber, low-fat diet is the ticket to feeling good and staying healthy.

Like cancer, the risk of *heart disease* is increased by a number of variables, among them smoking, alcohol use, weight, age, family history, and eating habits (see "Substance Abuse"). Luckily, you can control heart disease, too. Though you may think worrying about heart disease now is unnecessary, research shows that cholesterol builds up in the arteries of some children. That's serious when you consider the large amounts of cholesterol-heavy foods they may eat in the years to come.

How can you remedy this? You can reduce your risk for heart disease at the same time you are reducing your risk for cancer by eating a low-fat, low-cholesterol, low-sugar, and even low-sodium diet. Here's why:

• *Fat and cholesterol* cause your arteries to thicken, hindering the blood's ability to reach the heart. If a vessel carrying blood to the heart becomes blocked, a heart attack may occur.

• When you eat more *fat* or *sugar* than your body needs, the excess is changed to body fat. Excess weight helps fat-clogged arteries and high blood pressure to develop.

• When too much *salt* or *sodium* accumulates in the body fluids, the body tries to draw water out to balance things. This increases the blood volume and thus complicates high blood pressure. High blood pressure, in turn, increases the risk of heart disease. You may not have a problem with high blood pressure now, but it's a good idea to get used to a low-sodium diet as you may develop high blood pressure later.

(Other heart disease-related topics can be found in "Substance Abuse"; "Stress and Mental Health"; and "Exercise".)

Other less common diseases—osteoporosis, diabetes, and scurvy—have a lot to do with nutrition. But the general rule for all good health seems to be: Include all the basic food groups (low-fat dairy foods; fruits and vegetables; whole-grain breads and cereals; and lean meat, fish, poultry, and legumes) in your diet, and eat *everything* in moderation.

The Difference Between Fat on Your Stomach and Fat on Your Plate

Everybody has body fat; it helps cushion our organs and protect us from the cold. Some people have a lot of body fat (you usually can tell when it's too much), some have very little.

In this book we'll be most concerned about dietary fat—the kind in the food on your plate. What's interesting is that when there's too much fat in your diet (dietary fat) it can lead to too much fat in your body (body fat). (For an explanation, see "What's a Calorie?" page 32, and "Exercise: The Role it Plays in Diet," page 102.)

A lot of different foods have some dietary fat, but a few have a high-fat ratio: meats, dairy foods, oils, and butters. Those are the ones you have to watch out for. In some cases, dietary fat is easy to see and eliminate—like the skin on chicken and the gel on red meat. With other foods, you'll have to look for hidden fat and select low-fat types. The chart on this page should help.

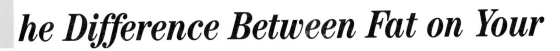

	HIGH-FAT Food Choices	LOW-FAT Alternatives
Dairy Foods	Whole milk Heavy cream Ice cream Most hard cheeses Sour cream	Skim milk Buttermilk Low-fat yogurt Ice milk Mozzarella made from part-skim milk Low-fat cottage cheese and ricotta cheese, low-fat plain yogurt
Meats	Sausage Corned beef Luncheon meats Ground beef Rib eye steak Liver	Lean boiled ham Flank steak London broil Lean ground beef Sirloin tip Veal
Poultry	With skin	Without skin
Fish	Smoked fish Canned fish packed in oil	Most fresh fish Canned fish packed in water

alcium for the Bones

Have you ever noticed that it seems easy for older women to fracture their hips? Or that some have a hump on their backs, at the top of the spine? Or that they get a little shorter as they get older? These are all symptoms of osteoporosis, a gradual loss and weakening of the bone structure. Even though it currently affects one in every four women, osteoporosis isn't something that you will suffer from now. Most women don't even see signs of it until after they stop menstruating (see "Menopause," and "Human Sexuality"), sometime in their late forties or early fifties. Still, research shows that *now*, during your teen years, is the best time to fortify yourself with calcium to prevent osteoporosis. This mineral is essential for strong bones. Drinking alcohol and smoking (see "Substance Abuse"), as well as lack of exercise (see "Exercise") also increase the risk of osteoporosis.

Some good calcium sources are low-fat milk, yogurt, and other dairy products; seafoods such as sardines, salmon, and oysters; dark green, leafy vegetables such as spinach, lettuce, and broccoli; almonds; and tofu.

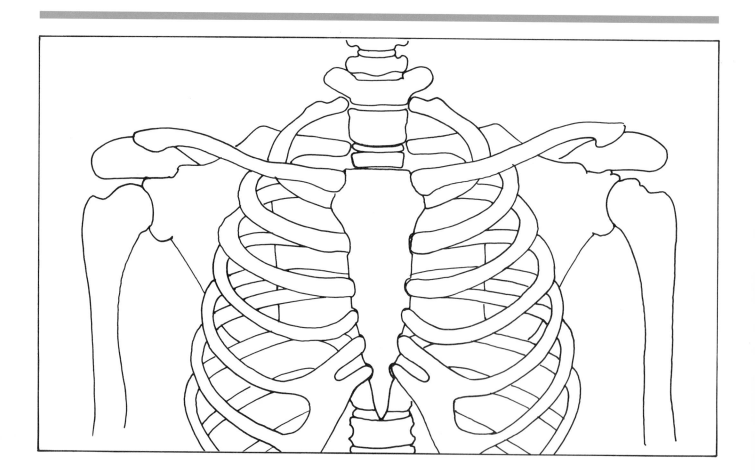

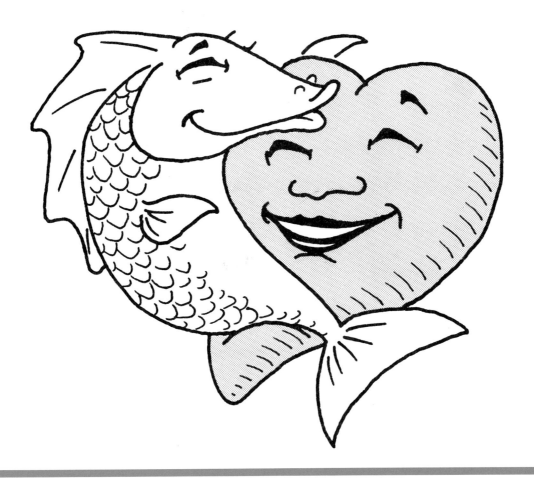

ish for the Heart:

It's Good Dietary Fat

Research shows that the dietary fat in cold water fish such as mackeral, salmon, sardines, or other oily fish, now called Omega-3, may prevent heart attacks. It seems that Eskimos and Japanese fishermen who eat seafood daily, hardly ever have heart problems. Since they first noticed this apparent correlation, scientists have done studies to prove it. Although the research isn't complete yet, it seems fish fat may have this effect because it thins blood and lowers cholesterol. And high cholesterol levels, as you know, cause heart problems by clogging up the veins. One note: those fish oil pills you see advertised have not yet been proven effective; your best bet is fresh fish.

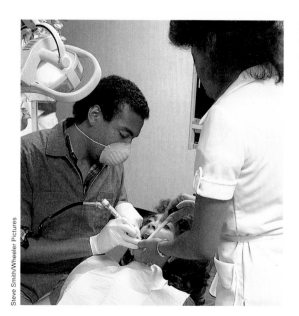

Sticky, sugary foods promote dental problems, but foods rich in calcium and vitamin D help make teeth and bones stronger.

Steve Smith/Wheeler Pictures

Growth

When you were younger your mother probably always told you to drink your milk so you'll grow up to be big and strong. And now, though you're nearly full-grown, you *should* still be drinking your milk (just make sure it's low-fat or skim milk) and eating well-rounded meals. Though you might not get any taller, your body will never completely stop growing. Regardless of age, the body is still going through everyday growing processes: Injuries heal, hair grows, new skin cells replace dead cells, and so on. Besides, you're shifting from childhood to adulthood and your body needs all the nutrients it can get to make those changes correctly. Also, a severe nutritional deficiency could delay puberty. And because these hormonal changes take so much energy, you need to be feeling your best. Eat well to feel well.

Appearance

Looks may be a little too important in our society, but none-the-less, they do matter. It's not to your advantage to be overly concerned with appearance, but healthy good looks are a reflection of a healthy body and a healthy self-image.

You've often heard that teeth are directly af-

fected by nutrition. If you grew up with a diet low in calcium and vitamin D, your teeth may not be as strong as they should be, since these nutrients are teeth-strengthening. Sticky, sugary foods, on the other hand, promote cavities, so avoid caramels, toffee, raisins, and similar foods. Follow all your dentist's advice too: Brush and floss after every meal.

Your complexion and hair are affected by both your body changes and eating habits. While you are developing into a man or a woman, hormones may be making your skin and hair oilier. You can't do too much about that, but you can control your diet to help keep you looking your best. Here's how:

• Drink plenty of water for livelier-looking skin and hair. Eight glasses a day is the minimum.

• Load up on fruits and vegetables. Not only do they contain an ample supply of water, they're also rich in the vitamins fundamental to healthy skin and hair.

• Because hair is made up of protein, protein-rich foods are also important to the diet. Be sure, however, to eat other good-for-looks foods as well. If you eat a lot of protein you're likely to be overloading on fat, since most protein foods are high in fat.

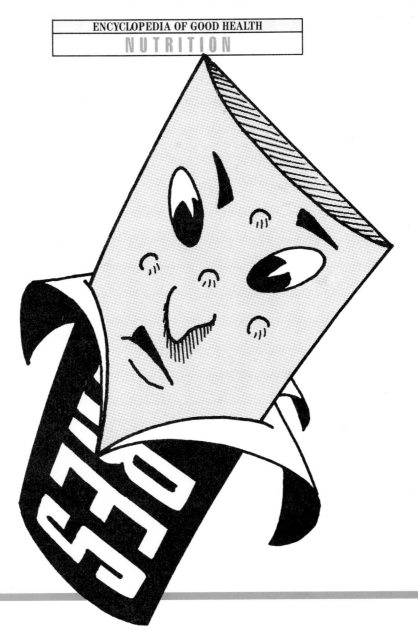

True or False?

Chocolate bars and French fries cause pimples.

A few years ago, we thought we could say "definitely true" to this statement. Now, we're not so sure. Some studies clearly show that greasy, sugary foods do *not* cause acne. On the other hand, some people swear that a certain food causes them to sprout pimples.

More than likely, puberty's overactive oil glands, poor hygiene, or stress causes this problem. But it doesn't hurt to cut down on high-fat foods like nuts, candy, cakes, pepperoni pizza, and other so-called "flare-up" foods.

Size

People who don't eat correctly could turn out to be underweight or overweight. Today, weight is a big concern to many people, as well as the cause of many problems. In some cases, people can't seem to keep their weight down to an ideal level. Others believe they're overweight when they're not. The most important thing to remember is that there's an ideal weight for everyone, and yours is based on your height and bone size—not on how big your brother or best friend is. You can

probably judge what size is right for you, but if there is any question, a doctor will tell you. Also, because good nutrition is even more important for you now, during puberty, it's best not to take on any weight-gain or weight-loss programs without a doctor's guidance (see "Good Reasons *Not* to Try to Lose Weight," page 69).

Besides, by following a healthy diet you shouldn't have to be too concerned about your size. In this case, it's more important for you to monitor your eating for the sake of health—not so you can be thinner than your best friend.

There is no "right" height and weight for girls or boys like you. Only your doctor can tell if you are under- or over-sized; but, if you want to get an idea of what's average, this chart should help. If it seems that you are far above or below average, check with your doctor. He or she will probably tell you not to worry and that there is a big difference in size among people your age.

Find your age and height on the chart. Each of the blue lines indicates how many kids your age are that tall or shorter.

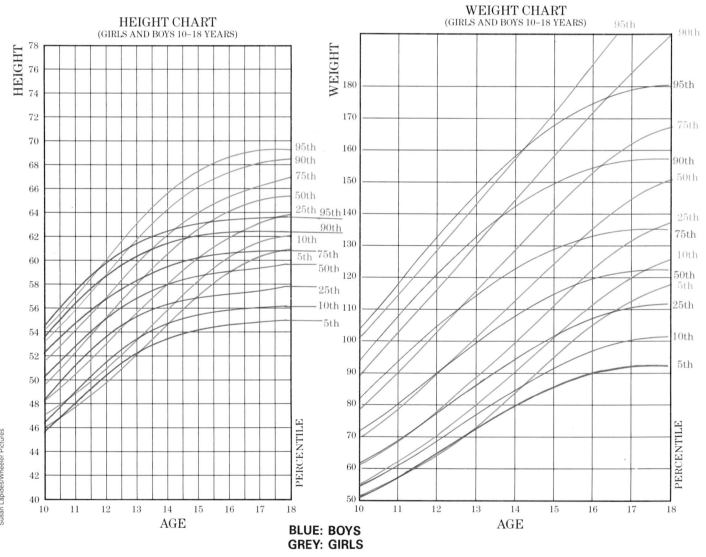

HEIGHT CHART
(GIRLS AND BOYS 10–18 YEARS)

WEIGHT CHART
(GIRLS AND BOYS 10–18 YEARS)

BLUE: BOYS
GREY: GIRLS

Susan Lapides/Wheeler Pictures

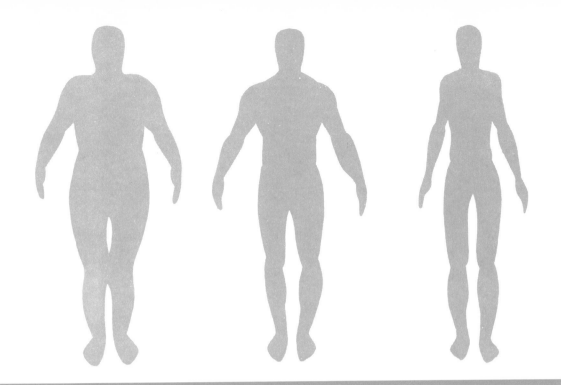

he Body Trap

Which body type best describes you?

As you can see, each shape above differs from the others. The endomorph is rounder and fuller all over. The smaller-boned ectomorph isn't necessarily thinner, but has a more narrow build. The more muscular mesomorph is somewhere in between.

A scientific theory holds that everyone leans toward one of these shapes. Just as you can't change your shoe size, you can't change the basic makeup of your body. All the dieting in the world won't turn the endomorph into an ectomorph, or vice versa. Likewise, all the dieting in the world won't make some stomachs positively flat. Some things we're born with—like height and body build.

That's not to say that an overweight person is predestined to be overweight. The weight-loss plan has a very important place within the realm of healthy habits—for people who really need it. Unfortunately, our society has gone overboard on the quest for thinness (see "When Thin is Dangerous" page 24). It's easy to be over-concerned and unrealistic about your body image. In fact, the ideal size (particularly for women) changes with the times. During the Great Depression, women were considerably rounder than they are now—and it was fashionable. These days, thin people are admired, but in other cultures—especially impoverished ones—to be plump is to be elite and beautiful.

The lesson: Don't fall into the "body trap" by overdieting and trying to change what is naturally yours. Stay at your ideal weight with healthy eating habits. Be happy with your body and realistic about what it can be. Make a *healthy* body your priority, and good looks will follow. Health is always in style.

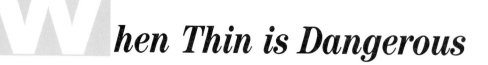

When Thin is Dangerous

Social standards and fashion have a lot to do with developing a person's body image. For some of us, keeping up with the times means cutting back on a few calories and increasing exercise a bit. For others, the desire to be thin is a much more serious ordeal. The result: eating disorders and illnesses that cause health problems for increasing numbers of people—90 percent of them girls and women.

Anorexia nervosa is one such eating disorder. This psychological illness causes a person to lose her appetite. She does all that she can to keep from eating, but when she does eat, she feels guilty. Oftentimes, the anorectic person loses so much weight that she looks and feels bad. Yet, she won't believe she looks sick when her friends or parents tell her so. Instead, she may think everyone is jealous of her thinness and attempting to sabotage her.

While the anorectic person is preoccupied with food and eating, her obsession is *caused* by other problems. It could be anger, fear, depression, or other emotional conditions. Often, the eating disorder arises when she tries to lose just a few pounds. When she does, she still feels "fat" and continues to cut back on food. Sometimes, she even relies on laxatives or purging (vomiting) to lose weight. By exercising extreme control over her eating habits, the anorectic individual thinks she is better able to deal with her emotional problems, but in the long run, the lack of nutrition puts her at an unhealthy disadvantage.

Bulimia is a related disorder. Like anorexia, bulimia is a fear of obesity. The illness is influenced by emotional disturbances, too. Yet, the bulimic person reacts by eating huge amounts of food (binging)—maybe 5,000 calories or more per day—and then taking laxatives or forcing herself to vomit. Ashamed of her eating patterns (the bulimic person believes what she is doing is abnormal, but the anorectic individual doesn't), people afflicted with bulimia may keep this binge-purge-binge cycle a secret from friends and family. Unfortunately, it's not always easy to tell that a person is bulimic, since she is often at a normal weight or slightly above.

If someone suffering from these eating disorders does not seek help, the result can be devastating. The anorectic person will eventually suffer from malnutrition—nutrient starvation—which leads to serious illnesses. A young person's growth may even be affected. The bulimic person, who loses important minerals every time she purges, can damage her heart and eventually experience a heart attack. What's more, strong acid from her stomach can damage her esophagus (mouth-to-stomach tube) and teeth.

How can you tell if a friend has these problems? Look for:

○ Puffy cheeks. Since the salivary glands are involved every time a person vomits, they become swollen. This could be a bulimic sign.
○ Deteriorating or yellowed teeth—another bulimic warning.
○ Bad breath—a result of purging.

○ Drastic weight losses—to the point where she doesn't look good.

○ Other appearance changes—pallid skin; dull, thinning hair.

○ Habitual after-meal trips to the bathroom.

○ Unusual eating patterns. If you notice a friend eating nothing but gum or skipping meals too frequently, it's cause for concern.

○ Avoidance of social outings. Bulimics may pass up a restaurant meal, because a trip to the bathroom is too obvious. Anorectic people simply don't want to be in an eating situation.

○ Distorted body images. A friend insists she's still got a few pounds to go when she's clearly below average weight.

○ Extreme exercising. Anorectic people may use heavy-duty workouts like they use laxatives and purging to lose weight.

For help and more information, contact:

American Anorexia/Bulimia Association, Inc. (AA/BA)
133 Cedar Lane
Teaneck, New Jersey 07666
(201) 836-1800
or
Anorexia Nervosa and Related Eating Disorders, Inc. (ANRED)
P.O. Box 5102
Eugene, Oregon 97405
(503) 344-1144
or
National Anorexic Aid Society, Inc. (NAAS)
P.O. Box 29461
Columbus, Ohio 43229
(614) 846-2588

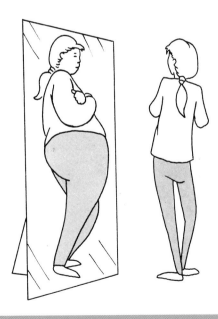

verweight is Probably Not...

...*Gaining three pounds* (a kilo) from one day to the next. On some days, your body tissue may hold more fluid than others.

...*Going up a size in clothes.* You're still growing and your body is changing. For an adult, this could be a sign, but not necessarily for you.

...*Weighing more than your friends.* Once again, your ideal weight is determined by your own frame and height—not by those of others.

...*Having a "flabby" stomach or "fat" legs.* These could be signs, but not necessarily. A doctor can tell you for sure. For one thing, puberty is changing your body dimensions, so maybe you're not used to the new you. Plus, we aren't always the best judge of how we look, but, at the same time, it's easy to be influenced by what others say.

verweight Could Be . . .

...*A big gain* of ten pounds (three or four kilos) or more in six months or less.

...*New clothes that don't fit*—even though they did when you got them.

...*Your mother or father worrying* that you are gaining too much too fast. They're not likely to mislead you. Plus, they can judge you from a distance.

...*Not being able to keep up* with your friends. When you're running or playing ball, do you feel "weighed down"? Do you think you're limited by your size? See a doctor if you're concerned.

Food is made up of elements that do different jobs.

"Vitamin A" and "protein" might not look like much on paper, but they mean a lot to your body on a daily basis. Different foods are teeming with different nutrients. Take a carrot, for example. You'll often hear it referred to as a "complex carbohydrate," but it contains a lot more than carbohydrates. There is also a little bit of protein, calcium, iron, thiamine, riboflavin, vitamin C, and a whopping dose of vitamin A.

If you aren't getting enough vitamins and minerals, your body will let you know. See "Energy and Performance" on page 12, and "What Really Happens When You Don't Eat" on page 15.

Here and on the following pages, we'll show you how all those nutrients and vitamins work on and with your body.

Six Different Food Groups

1. Carbohydrates (simple and complex)
2. Protein
3. Fat
4. Vitamins
5. Minerals
6. Water

Carbohydrates

Definition: Made up of sugar and starches.

Purpose: To provide energy for the body.

Good points: The carbohydrate group includes the natural complex carbohydrates (see below).

Bad points: Many of today's carbohydrates have little starch but lots of sugar, such as cake and sugar-coated cereals.

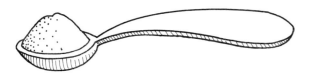

Simple Carbohydrates (Sugar)

Definition: The sweet-tasting substance found naturally in some foods, such as milk and fruit. You can't see those sugars. The kind you can see—like white and brown sugar—have been refined, or changed from natural sugars.

Purpose: To give you quick energy. Sugar is simple enough so that it's ready to enter your bloodstream and feed your cells more quickly than other foods.

Good points: Except for the "bad points" below, sugar seems to cause no problems for the body.

Bad points: (1) Sugars themselves only give the body calories; they have no vitamins, minerals, or fiber. (2) Because sugar is usually found in fatty foods like cake and candy, it can indirectly cause obesity and heart disease.

Complex Carbohydrates (Starch)

Definition: These carbohydrates are found in foods derived from plants, like potatoes, beans, corn, bread, pasta, and cereal. They provide the body with vitamins, minerals, fiber, and calories.

Purpose: Like sugar, complex carbohydrates are the body's main source of energy.

Good points: For very few calories, they're loaded with nutrients (see "What's a Calorie?" page 32).

Bad points: Actually, complex carbohydrates are the only major nutrient not known to have any long-term risks.

Carbohydrates

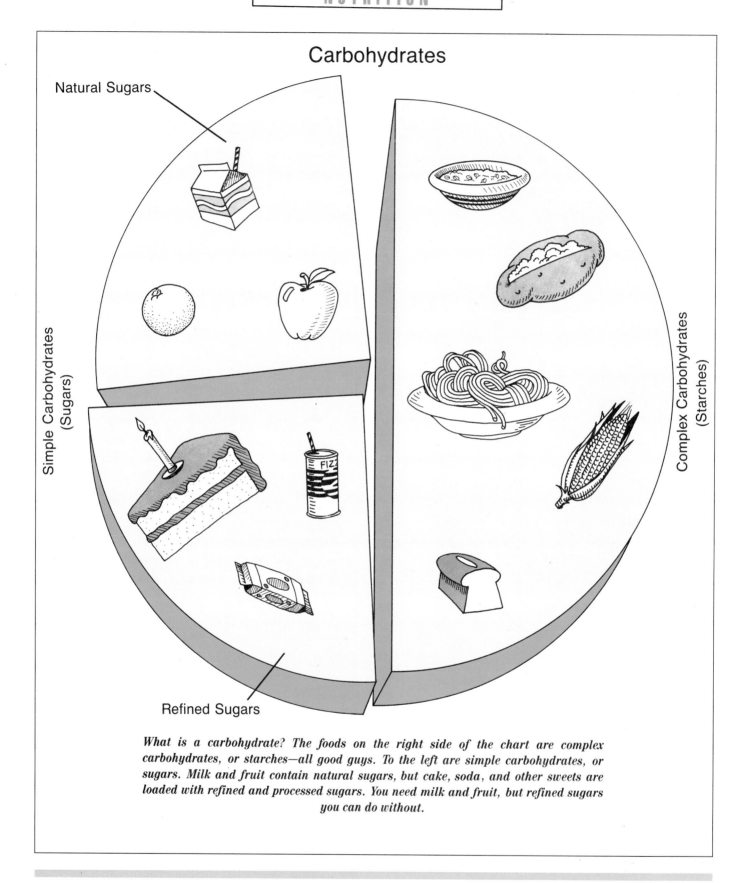

Natural Sugars

Simple Carbohydrates (Sugars)

Refined Sugars

Complex Carbohydrates (Starches)

What is a carbohydrate? The foods on the right side of the chart are complex carbohydrates, or starches—all good guys. To the left are simple carbohydrates, or sugars. Milk and fruit contain natural sugars, but cake, soda, and other sweets are loaded with refined and processed sugars. You need milk and fruit, but refined sugars you can do without.

Sugar Smarts

- 70 percent of the sugar in our diet is hidden in processed foods, such as cereal, ketchup, peanut butter, and soda.
- Every person eats an average of 130 pounds (about 48 kilos) of sugar every year—an average of thirty-six teaspoons of sugar everyday.
- Nine teaspoons of sugar go into a twelve-ounce (360-milliliters) can of soda.
- You could totally do without the refined sugar in your sugar bowl. Instead, the body could use the natural sugars found in natural foods.

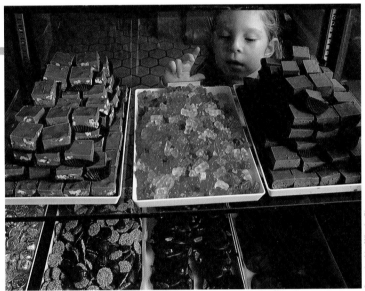

Susan Lapides/Wheeler Pictures

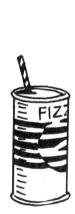 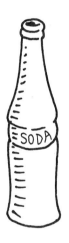

True or False?

Starches, or complex carbohydrates, make you fat.

At one time, everybody *thought* baked potatoes, corn, pasta, beans, and other starchy foods were fattening and bad for us. Now we know that complex carbohydrates have more nutrition and fewer calories than any other food group. That's not to say you can eat piles of pasta without gaining weight, but you should make starchy foods a big part of your meals.

Substituting Sugar

Wouldn't it be great if all those high-fat, high-sugar, disease-causing, obesity-triggering foods could be substituted with perfectly safe, just-as-good-tasting look-alikes?

Thanks to high-technology, the day may come when we *can* have German chocolate cake without the fat and sugar. In the meantime, we've got artificial sweeteners, such as aspartame, a substance that's 200 times sweeter than sugar with 95 percent fewer calories. Then there's saccharin, a white powder that's 300 times sweeter than sugar and, also, extremely low in calories.

With these two dynamos on our side, you might think all our sweet-tooth problems would be solved. But it's not that easy. In some cases, artificial sweeteners have made life easier. Diet sodas with aspartame, for example, give you the sweet taste of a carbonated drink without sugar. In many restaurants, saccharin is available along with sugar for coffee and tea.

Then, there are the drawbacks. At one time, saccharin was banned from the market after it caused bladder tumors in animal research. Because it couldn't be proven that saccharin caused cancer in *humans*, it's back on the market. As for aspartame, it's been proven safe for most individuals time and time again (see "Cholesterol, Sodium, and Additives," page 46). Yet, many consumer groups still believe it causes problems for unborn babies and others.

Aspartame and saccharin are also limited in their uses. To some people, saccharin leaves behind an unpleasant aftertaste. Aspartame loses its flavor at high temperatures, so aspartame-sweetened baked foods are out. Other sugar substitutes on the market have their problems, too. For example, sugar-free gums often contain sorbitol, mannitol, or xylitol, but, unfortunately, these are not low-calorie sweeteners. In fact, they have about the same number of calories as sugar.

Should you be concerned about artificial sweeteners? Don't think that because they are substitutes, you can eat as much of them as you would like. Once again, the rule, "everything in moderation," applies. In all the sugar substitute tests, scientists found that small amounts of these substances didn't cause problems. A diet soda or a saccharin-sweetened tea each day is probably safe. However, if you find that you're particularly sensitive to these products (for example, you always develop a headache after drinking diet soda), it might be wise to check with a doctor or completely exclude the substitute from your diet.

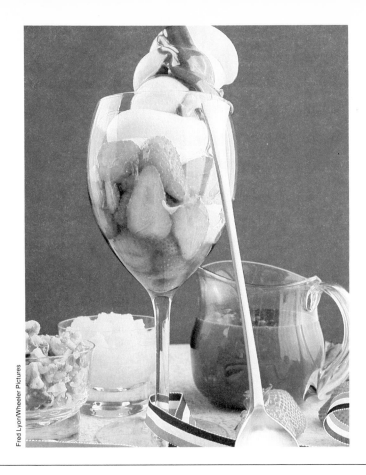

Although this sundae looks scrumptious, it won't seem so appealing when its nutritional content is revealed. First of all, don't be fooled by the fruit and nuts into thinking that this is a good-for-you food. Their value is canceled by the 14 teaspoons of sugar in the ice cream and fudge sauce. Now, take a look at the calories, fat content, cholesterol tally, and sodium count below.

	Calories	Fat (g)	Cholesterol (mg)	Sodium (mg)
Ice cream, 1 cup (200 grams)	270	14	60	120
Fudge sauce, 3 tablespoons (2 British tablespoons)	150	1.5		30
Strawberries, ½ cup (100 grams)	140			3
Pineapple, ½ cup (100 grams)	95			3
Walnuts, ¼ cup (50 grams)	160	16		
Total	815	31.5	60	156

This analysis shows that a hot fudge sundae is loaded with calories, sugar, and fat, without the benefits of good-for-you elements like protein and fiber—at least not enough to be worth the fat and calorie intake. Though you probably won't make a chart like this for every food you eat, try to do a quick analysis in your head of the costs and rewards of each food before you eat it.

What's a Calorie?

A. A calorie is a measurement of how much energy a food produces; that's the technical definition. Most of us tend to think of a calorie as something that makes us fat. Reason: When we eat too many calories, the body can't use them all. The excess is stored in fat cells. Only carbohydrates, proteins, and fats in the food you eat can make calories—not nutrients such as vitamin A or calcium.

 What's an Empty Calorie?

A. That's the term used for foods with plenty of calories but no nutrients. For example, a medium-sized baked potato has 100 calories, and lots of nutrients such as vitamin C, protein, iron, phosphorous, and more. But six ounces of soda also has 100 calories mostly in sugar but little else. Nutrition experts call foods with lots of sugar— also called simple carbohydrates—and few nutrients, empty calories.

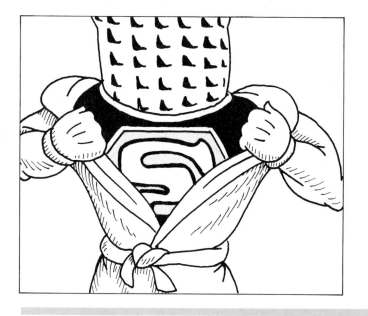

Fiber: Super Food!

If there's one nutrition word you've heard before, it's likely to be fiber. What is fiber? It is the material from plant cells that gives plants their structure. We can eat it, but we can't completely digest it, and that's why it's good for you. By bulking up and speeding the waste out of your body, fiber improves digestion and cuts down the risk of cancer. Though doctors aren't sure why, some studies also show that fiber helps lower blood pressure and cholesterol levels. Plus, it's good for weight control, since fiber-rich foods are filling and low in calories.

While Americans eat only about ten to twenty grams of fiber a day, doctors recommend that we eat around twice that—the amount found in a bowl of high-fiber bran cereal, an apple with skin, two slices of whole wheat bread from a sandwich, and a bran muffin. Below, we've listed some good fiber sources. Notice that these are complex carbohydrates: fruits, vegetables, and whole grains. And remember: When you're eating a lot of fiber, it's important to drink plenty of liquids to help move them out of the body.

- Whole-grain crackers
- Apples
- Pinto beans
- Carrots
- Whole-grain bagels
- Bananas
- Shredded wheat cereal
- Bran muffins
- Pumpernickel bread
- Oranges
- Whole-grain cereal
- Lima beans
- Corn
- Sweet potatoes
- Corn bread
- Whole-grain pasta

Whenever possible, eat foods in their freshest state, for a bigger dose of nutrients. Less (or no) cooking means more fiber, too, because cooking breaks down the plant walls in food, which is the "roughage" that's so essential.

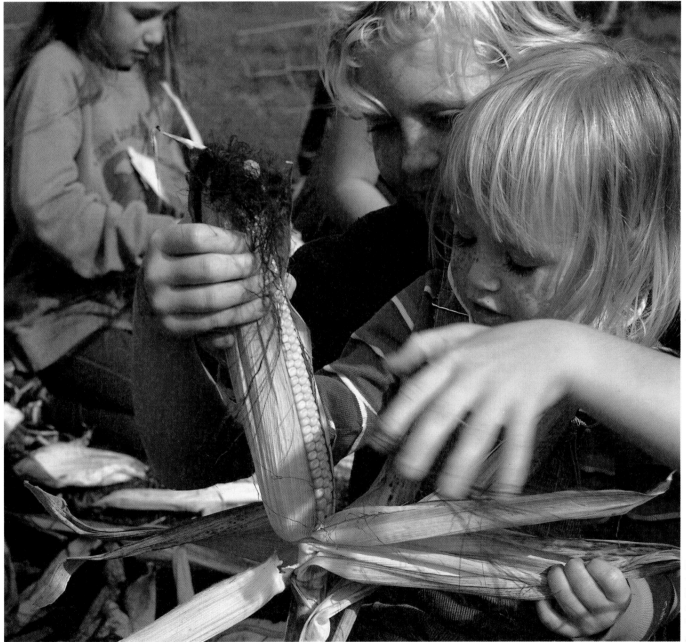

Susan Lapides/Wheeler Pictures

What's a Whole Grain?

A. A whole grain is a plant food in which the kernel is whole. The kernel has three parts: the endosperm, the germ, and the bran. Most of the grains we eat, such as white flour or white rice, have one or two of the parts removed—they've been refined. This lowers the amount of nutrients you get from them. A loaf of white bread labeled "enriched" means the makers added back some of those missing nutrients, but not all of them.

How can you tell if a product is whole grain or not? Look for :

○ Hot and cold cereals, such as shredded wheat, oatmeal, and bran. You can usually tell if they're whole grain by reading the label.
○ Breads labeled "whole wheat." "Wheat" bread isn't always the same thing.
○ Pumpernickel, rye, and corn breads.
○ Muffins, pizza dough, and even cakes and cookies can be made with whole-grain flours, but some aren't easy to find. Ask your grocer for some or visit a health-food store.
○ Whole-wheat pasta, pancakes, and waffles.
○ Brown rice.

"Refined" or "Processed" Means...

...A food is not in its most natural state. The food has been changed by machine or chemicals. Example: A red, shiny apple is natural, but the apple in an apple snack cake has been processed. Often the flavor in a packaged food isn't real. It's been made to taste like apple with other substances. Another example: Table sugar doesn't grow out of the ground in white crystals. It's made, or refined, from sugarcane or sugar beets through a chemical or mechanical process. Processed foods in and of themselves are not bad for you, but the heavily processed foods usually maintain little nutrient value and could be classified as empty calories. On the other hand, the words natural or organic on the label do not insure that the contents are healthy.

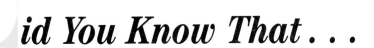

id You Know That...

...When the body doesn't get enough carbohydrates, it has to rely solely on protein for energy. As a result, there's not enough protein for building and repairing cells. In fact, until adulthood, protein is absolutely essential for normal body growth.

Protein

Definition: Substance in meat, fish, poultry, dairy foods, dried beans and peas (legumes), egg whites, and nuts.

Purpose: To build and repair all tissues in the body, to provide energy, and to fight infection.

Good points: Most sources of protein are nutritious in other ways as well. Legumes are complex carbohydrates. Dairy foods have calcium and vitamin D. Meat and fish contain a wealth of other minerals and vitamins, too.

Bad points: Some protein sources, such as various meat and dairy products, are also high in fat. As a result, protein-heavy diets have been connected to high blood pressure and cholesterol levels.

True or False?

Athletes should load up on protein.

False. Football coaches have been known to push steak after steak at their players, believing the extra protein would build their muscles. Proteins are *necessary* for muscles to work, but they don't *build* them—exercise does. In fact, a high-protein diet might do more harm to muscles than good. Red meat is often high in fat, which causes cholesterol to build up in the arteries. This way, blood has a harder time of reaching the muscles, which slows down their development.

Fat

Definition: Substance found in nuts, meats, oils, eggs, chocolate, margarine, olives, dairy foods, and so on.

Purpose: To supply the most concentrated fuel for the body, to help the body absorb important vitamins, to insulate the body, and to cushion organs.

Good points: Adds flavor to many foods.

Bad points: Fat has been linked to cancer, heart disease, strokes, and obesity.

The Many Faces of Fat

What's the difference? Some are worse than others.

Saturated fats are usually found in all meats and in dairy products such as butter, and cheese. (These fats are also found in a very limited number of vegetable products such as palm oil, coconut oil, and palm kernel oil.) This fat causes the most problems, since it tends to increase cholesterol in the blood.

Polyunsaturated fats are found mostly in specific plant foods such as vegetable oil, corn oil, and margarine. Although research shows that in small amounts these fats can lower the blood cholesterol, it's always best to limit all fats. These fats are better for you than the saturated fats.

Monosaturated fats include peanut, olive, and rice oils. Supposedly, they have little effect on cholesterol. Whenever you have a choice select these fats or no fats at all.

This information will help you to make healthier food choices. Example: If you were going to make an omelet, would you put butter or vegetable oil in the skillet? What oil is best for salad dressing—olive or vegetable? Monosaturated fats (peanut, olive, and rice oils) are better than polyunsaturated and saturated fats; polyunsaturated fats are better than saturated fats.

Fat Fact

Nutritionally speaking, we need to eat only one tablespoon (15 milliliters) of polyunsaturated fat each day. *However,* the average American eats six to eight times that much fat every time he drinks a glass of whole milk.

True or False?

Vitamin E cures warts.

False. Not only does it not cure warts, vitamin E isn't the answer to wrinkles, ulcers, arthritis, cancer, or heart disease. A lot of people make a lot of claims about vitamin E, but no nationally recognized medical experts in this area have agreed with them.

WHERE FATS ARE FOUND

Use this chart to find which kinds of fat are found in which foods. Remember that saturated fats are usually solid at room temperature and come primarily from animal sources. Both polyunsaturated fats and monounsaturated fats come from specific vegetable sources. It's tricky to remember which fats are better for you. Study the chart, then try to cut back on saturated and polyunsaturated fats. Of course, it's best to cut back on all fats if you can.

KIND OF FAT	EXAMPLES	
Saturated	Butter Beef Cheese Chocolate Coconut Coconut oil	Egg yolk Milk Palm oil Poultry Vegetable shortening
Polyunsaturated	Almonds Corn oil Cottonseed oil Fish Margarine	Mayonnaise Pecans Safflower oil Soybean oil Sunflower oil
Monounsaturated	Avocado Cashews Olives Olive oil	Peanuts Peanut oil Peanut butter

Vitamins

Definition: Substances that don't provide energy but are important for other body functions.

Purpose: To help the body use energy and nutrients from food, and to help make blood.

Good points: They're abundant in natural foods.

Bad points: Like anything, you can get too many vitamins, leading to harmful results (see "Everything in Moderation," page 47).

True or False?

Vitamin C chases away colds.

True and **False.** By having enough vitamin C and other vitamins in your diet, your body might be able to fight off a cold. But vitamins can't make a cold go away after you've caught it.

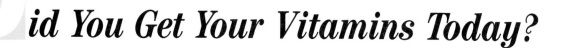

Did You Get Your Vitamins Today?

Remember those colored, cartoon-shaped vitamins that Mom or Dad gave you when you were little? They probably weren't necessary. Vitamins that don't come directly from the foods you eat are called supplements; they've been artificially made. They work in your body, but any doctor will tell you that foods are better sources of vitamins.

In some cases, a doctor might recommend a supplement in addition to a vitamin-rich diet. For example, calcium and iron are sometimes hard to get enough of in foods. Then, of course, you'll want to do what your doctor recommends.

VITAMIN	FUNCTION	BEST SOURCES
A	Needed for growth; promotes healthy eyes, skin, and linings of the throat and digestive tract.	Dark yellow, orange, and dark green vegetables and fruits, such as spinach and cantaloupe; eggs; low-fat cheese.
B includes four different kinds:		
B1 or Thiamine	Needed for the nervous system (what causes you to react when you put your hand on a hot stove); helps the body get energy from food.	Ham; oysters; whole-grain and enriched cereals, pasta, and bread; oatmeal; peas and lima beans.
B2 or Riboflavin	Good for the skin; helps the body use oxygen.	Dark green vegetables; eggs; whole-grain and enriched breads, pasta, and cereals; mushrooms; dried legumes; skim milk; low-fat meat.
Niacin	Same as B1 and B2	Same as B1 and B2
B6	Helps body absorb protein.	Whole-grain (but not enriched) cereals and breads; spinach; green beans; bananas; fish; poultry; potatoes.
B12	Helps the body use protein, fat, and carbohydrates, and make red blood cells (the carriers of oxygen to your body parts).	Only in animal foods: low-fat meat and milk; fish; oysters.
C	Helps keep gums healthy; holds the body cells together.	Citrus fruits; tomatoes; strawberries; potatoes; green peppers; other dark green vegetables.
D	Helps the body absorb calcium for strong bones and teeth.	Eggs; low-fat milk; salmon; tuna.
E	Helps make red blood cells, muscles, and other tissues; protects vitamin A.	Vegetable oils; whole-grain cereals and breads; dried beans; green, leafy vegetables.

Minerals

Definition: Substances that don't provide energy but perform other important functions for your body.

Purpose: They all have different jobs, but calcium, for example, helps to make bones. Potassium helps muscles to work. (See the chart on page 41).

Good points: Many are only needed in tiny amounts, so shortages are rare.

Bad points: Some people abuse supplements and take large doses of minerals (see "Did You Get Your Vitamins Today?," page 38). Unfortunately, a few (iron, zinc, fluoride) are poisonous in large amounts.

Stock up on these "power foods." They're high in vitamin A and C, which have been linked with lower risks of cancer.

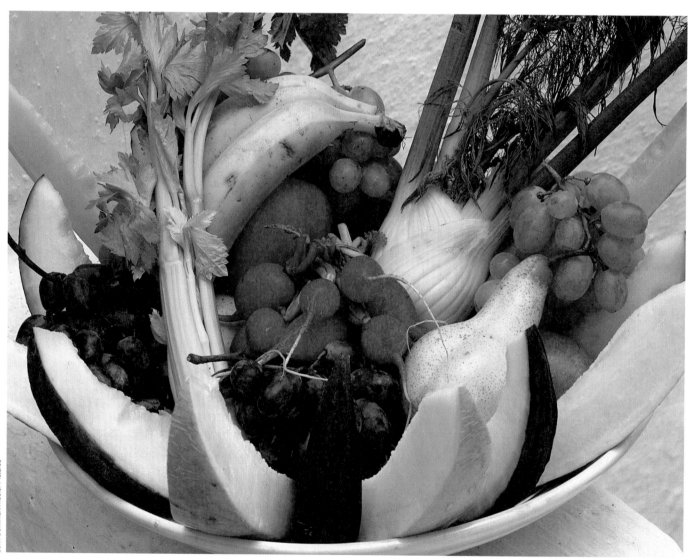

John Dominis/Wheeler Pictures

id You Know That...

...Around the turn of the century, some scientists experimented by feeding rats pure protein, carbohydrates, and fat because they were the only nutrients they knew about then. What happened? The rats died. Vitamins were missing from their diets.

MINERAL	FUNCTION	BEST SOURCES
The Most Important Minerals (Be conscientious about including these foods in your diet.)		
Calcium and phosphorous (If you're getting one, you're probably getting the other)	Supports growth and strength of bones and teeth; holds cells together; helps blood clot.	Low-fat dairy foods; sardines and canned salmon; green, leafy vegetables.
Iron	Helps blood carry oxygen through the body and release energy from food.	Whole-grains; eggs; low-fat meats; dried beans.
Fluoride	Prevents tooth decay; may also prevent loss of bone structure with age.	Fish; tea; most low-fat animal foods.
The Others (Also necessary though most people get what they need without trying.)		
Magnesium	Helps nerves and muscles to function properly.	Nuts; low-fat meat; fish; whole grains.
Potassium	Helps muscles and the heart to function properly.	Bananas; oranges; dried fruits.
Copper	Helps blood do its job.	Nuts; cocoa powder; raisins; dried beans.
Iodine	Helps the thyroid gland function.	Seafood; table salt.
Zinc	Aids with appetite and growth.	Low-fat meat; eggs; seafood.
Chromium	Gives energy. Helps your body break down and use carbohydrates.	Whole grains; low-fat meats and cheese.

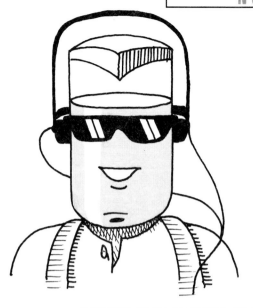

Water

Definition: The single most important food substance, available in liquids as well as in fruits and vegetables.

Purpose: To carry nutrients and waste through the body; to help keep body temperature even (through perspiration); to keep joints and muscles flexible.

Good points: If you drink more water than you need, the body simply gets rid of it through waste.

Bad points: The body doesn't do a good job of telling you how much water you need.

Water Wisdom

○ You could live weeks, maybe even a month, without food. But you wouldn't last three days without water.

○ As human beings, we're walking, talking water tanks. Your blood is 83 percent water; your brain, 75 percent.

○ Water is wonderful for making you look and feel your best. Drink a minimum of eight glasses a day for livelier hair and skin. It can even help reduce the number of wrinkles you may develop some day. Try water (a tall glass with a twist of lemon, or fruit-flavored sparkling water) instead of soda, and you'll be surprised by how much better you feel.

True or False?

Athletes should take salt tablets to replace the salt they lose in sweat.

False. Not only is the salt tablet unnecessary, it could be harmful. When the body perspires a great deal, it begins to make its own adjustments to replace lost salt. When you try to help it out with a dose of salt, the balance goes crazy. The result: Muscle contractions are affected, and the blood thickens, neither of which are desirable.

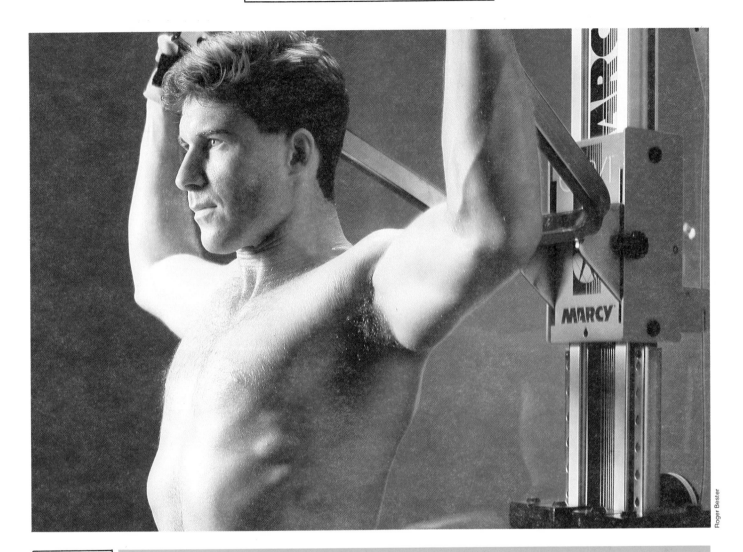

Roger Bester

True Or False?

Athletes should drink a lot of water to replace the water

they lose from sweating.

True. That's one thing you can't overdo. In fact, it's good to drink water both before and after exercise. What about the "thirst-quenching" athletic drinks? Water is even more beneficial.

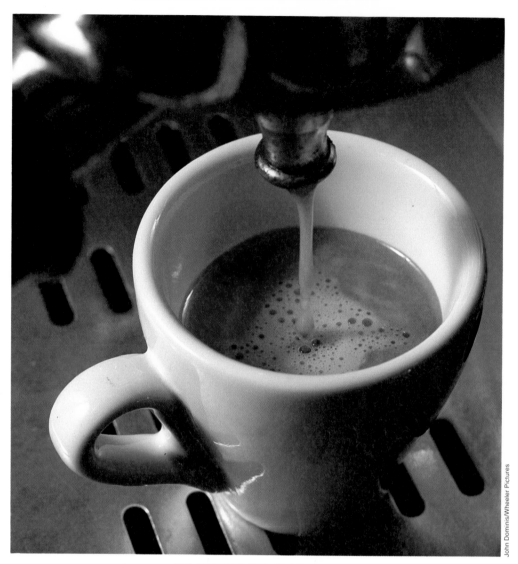

John Dominis/Wheeler Pictures

CAFFEINE COUNT

FOOD	CAFFEINE (mg)
Soft drinks (12 ounces)	50
Coffee	
Drip (5 ounces)	145
Percolated (5 ounces)	110
Instant, regular (5 ounces)	50
Decaffeinated (5 ounces)	2
Tea	
One-minute brew (5 ounces)	20
Three-minute brew (5 ounces)	30
Five-minute brew (5 ounces)	40
Cocoa and Chocolate	
Cocoa beverage (6 ounces)	10
Milk chocolate (1 ounce)	5
Baking chocolate (1 ounce)	35

The Caffeine Kick

Caffeine comes naturally from many different plants, but we know it as the uplifting substance in coffee, tea, soda, and chocolate. In our society, we rely on it as a stimulant—something to wake us up when we're sleepy.

Some studies even suggest that heavy coffee or caffeine consumption (we're not sure which is the culprit) leads to more serious health problems, such as bladder cancer, fibrocystic breast disease, and higher cholesterol levels. In most cases, these findings also involved smoking cigarettes and/or drinking several cups of coffee a day.

The doctors' general conclusion: Caffeine is certainly safer than most stimulants, but you have to keep it under control. The caffeine stopping point depends on your weight, age, health, and how you feel when you've had a lot of caffeine. Pregnant women, for example, have to be careful with caffeine because it tends to stay in their systems longer. In your case, particularly with all the growing and hormonal changes you're experiencing, you might feel better by taking it easy on caffeine. Stay away from the stay-awake pills available at the drugstore. Although a lot of students try to use them for late-night study sessions, these caffeine drugs usually make them feel ill and make concentrating even more difficult.

Cholesterol, Sodium, and Additives

The problem with these substances is that they're difficult to avoid or not harmful in small amounts, but most of us get too much of them. Unfortunately, cholesterol, sodium, and additives are the source of many problem diseases.

Cholesterol is a waxy, fat-like substance found only in foods from animals. It's not a fat, but it usually is distributed throughout fat—especially saturated fat. That's why animal-made fatty foods—meats, dairy foods, eggs—are high in cholesterol and saturated fat.

Cholesterol is generally considered to be unhealthy, but it's actually needed by the body. The liver itself produces cholesterol to help make cell membranes, hormones, vitamin D, and other essentials. The body makes as much cholesterol as it will ever need, and thus we do not need to consume it in the foods we eat.

Babies require additional cholesterol in their diets. Their bodies aren't developed enough to make all that they require. But as you get older, you don't really need any extra cholesterol. Never-the-less, the average American eats about 600 milligrams of cholesterol a day. As a result, the cholesterol builds in the arteries, interrupting the blood flow and damaging the heart. It's no wonder heart disease is our biggest killer!

Sodium is another food topic that is frequently debated. Generally, it's given a bad name, but salt, or sodium chloride, benefits the body, too. It regulates body fluid and helps nerve impulses to travel and the heart to beat. Salt comes not only from the salt shaker; trace amounts come from foods in their natural state. The rest we get from canned soups, canned vegetables, pickles, ketchup, cereal, and other packaged foods.

The problem with sodium is that we get too much of it. Doctors say we don't have to lay a hand on the salt shaker to get the 220 milligrams we need daily. However, most people take in more than that.

At first it was thought that high-sodium diets *caused* high blood pressure and heart problems. Recent evidence, however, suggests that it doesn't; low-sodium diets help control the condition in some people with high blood pressure.

What does this mean? Sodium is less of an issue for you (unless you know you have a blood pressure problem) and more of an issue for any of your relatives who have high blood pressure. This isn't to say you should ignore the salt in your diet, though. We can't be sure, but minimizing your salt intake may help prevent your blood pressure from going up later in life. So, it's wise to get in the low-sodium habit now. (For women only, see also "Especially for Women," page 75.)

Food additives are another vital topic of this nutrition discussion. Information about additives is often confusing.

The trouble is that additives aren't always unnatural or unnecessary. Many added "chemicals" are natural substances. Vitamin C, iron, and calcium, for example, often "fortify" packaged foods. Manufacturers also put additives in foods to improve taste or increase shelf life. Without additives, you can forget about frozen or canned foods. They wouldn't be too appetizing by the time they had traveled from the factory, to the supermarket, to the kitchen. So even when additives are people-made, they're often necessary.

However, some additives may do more harm than good. Those kinds have people wondering and worrying. In some cases, the government studies questionable additives. A few, like certain food dyes and artificial sweeteners, seem to increase cancer risk, so they have been restricted or completely banned. Others, like aspartame (a sugar substitute found in diet sodas), have been proven safe for now (see "Substituting Sugar," page 30.)

Unfortunately, the government can't afford the time and money it takes to answer all our questions about food additives fast enough. Years from now, you may find out that a food you never suspected and have been eating all your life is dangerous.

What can we do about it now? Avoid additives when you can by eating more fresh and frozen foods, as opposed to processed varieties. An extra precaution: Wash off fresh fruits and vegetables. A layer of insect-killing chemicals may have been left behind.

The Government's Watchdog

Whenever a new food product is developed, the government won't let it be marketed until it has been tested thoroughly. It often takes several years for the product to finally reach the supermarket.

There's a good reason for the thorough investigation. To make sure our foods and medicines do what they're supposed to do without danger, the government created the Food and Drug Administration (FDA). The FDA will make sure a substance doesn't have something harmful in it, then put it through long-term tests. If too many people complain that the product made them queasy, the FDA will whisk it back into the lab for more tests.

The FDA is an important force in our country. Some people think its rules are too strict; others think they are not strict enough. The truth is new ideas are approved all the time.

Everything in Moderation

Nutrients and vitamins do all kinds of great things for your body, but that doesn't mean you should consume too much of a particular food to get specific nutritional benefits. All the food sources described here are very important, but should be taken in moderate amounts. Too little calcium, as you know, can leave you with weak bones. But too much can make you drowsy and tired, or form calcium deposits where they don't belong. Neglect your vitamin A, and you might end up with a case of night blindness. But overload on vitamin A-rich carrots, and you could be rewarded with yellowing skin.

In our country, where we have a wide variety of foods to choose from, we generally manage to get all our vitamins. Still, you'll always be at your best by consciously working nutrients and vitamins into your diet. This can be accomplished by following a well-balanced eating plan. The "Take Charge!" section, pages 76-78, should help. How about two percent (lowfat) milk as an alternative? I'll bet you can hardly tell the difference from whole milk.

CHOLESTEROL COUNT

This chart will give you an idea of the amount of the cholesterol in some common foods.

	SERVING	CHOLESTEROL (mg)
Whole milk	1 cup	33
Cheese:		
Cheddar	1 oz	30
Cottage/creamed (4% fat)	1 cup	31
Swiss	1 oz	26
Light cream	1 Tbsp	10
Sour cream	1 Tbsp	5
Ice cream	1 cup	59
Yogurt, plain (part skim)	1 cup	14
Lean beef	3 oz	77
Poultry (flesh without skin, light meat)	3 oz	43
Fish	3 oz	43
Shrimp	11 large	96
Tuna (packed in oil, drained)	3 oz	55
Lobster	½ cup	62
Liver, beef	3 oz	372
Frankfurters (all beef-30% fat)	2 large	15
Eggs	1 medium	274
Peanut butter	2 Tbsp	0
Bacon, cooked crisp	2 slices	14
Butter	1 Tbsp	31
Imitation (diet) margarine	1 Tbsp	0
Mayonnaise	1 Tbsp	8

Society plays a big role in our eating habits.

After the school day is over, you and your friends may often head for a nearby fast-food restaurant.

As you talk with friends there, you probably don't pay much attention to what you are eating.

In the past, people gathered at a friendly barn raising or a chatter quilting bee. Today, most people socialize over food—it's a natural for our society. Most business and pleasure is done during meals. But this doesn't mean that you have to eat desserts and other unhealthy foods whenever the opportunity arises. For example, during the holiday season, your relatives may tempt you with home-baked desserts. Your family may also have a tradition of rewarding your achievements with food.

Even though fast-food restaurants are great places to relax after a hard day at school, your food choices in most social places aren't usually healthy. And it's not exactly easy to say no to a hot dog when everyone else is eating. By being aware of how socializing influences your eating you'll already be better off.

These are examples of how your family can influence your eating habits. Since the dawn of time, we've expressed love, sympathy, appreciation, pride, and other emotions with food. Some of us grow up thinking food is the answer or reward to everything until we develop a weight problem. It's pretty tough to unlearn such habits. So, it helps to realize what's happening.

Next to friends and family, keep an eye on advertisements, which often encourage the consumer to eat foods that are not necessarily nutritious. Advertising often makes false promises, too, leading you to believe that a product can benefit you more than it actually will.

Although commercials often fade into the background in the American home, their messages often get through to the consumer. We don't think about it too much, but we're definitely more aware of products we've seen advertised.

Remember though, that the people who produce advertisements are just doing their job: They're getting you to buy a product. They try to make the candy or restaurant or drink look as good as possible. There are many things they don't tell you, such as the fat content of fast food or the amount of sugar in some breakfast cereals.

More and more, you'll see healthier foods advertised. People are concerned about how foods are marketed—particularly how ad campaigns are meant to influence children and teens—so they're trying to change things. Still, you're the one who's in control, who has to decide what advertised food is or isn't worth eating. The best way to decide is to stay informed. In "How to Read a Food Label" on page 89 we tell you how to read a label. Ask your doctor or your health teacher if you have questions about which foods are best for you. Keep aware and you'll be fine and healthy.

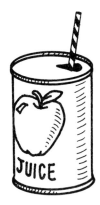

I.D. I. Q.

In the group below, identify which foods are highest in fat.

A. Soy sauce   B. Thousand Island dressing   C. Mayonnaise   D. Mustard

Mayonnaise is the hands-down winner with one tablespoon containing 11.2 grams of fat. Thousand Island dressing is second with one tablespoon containing 8.0 grams. Soy sauce may be high in sodium, but it and mustard are good next-to-no-fat condiments.

I.D. I.Q.

In the group below, identify which are highest in sodium.

A. Tomato juice   B. Apple juice   C. Tea   D. Diet soda

You could probably taste-test this question and get it right. Tomato juice is the saltier one: one cup has 880 milligrams of sodium. Diet soda has about thirty-nine milligrams. The other two foods are sodium-safe.

I.D. I.Q.

Identify which are the complex carbohydrates in the group below.

A. Hamburger   B. Pasta   C. Chicken   D. Fish

Pasta is the only complex carbohydrate in this group. Hamburger, chicken, and fish are proteins.

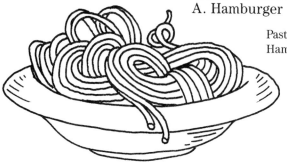

THE LEANEST MEATS

Healthy meat-eating begins with a wise choice of meat cut. Generally, the cuts with the lowest fat content come from the muscular parts of the animal, such as the shoulder or flank. Then, pick the piece with the least amount of marbling or white streaks of fat. Finally, before you cook the meat, trim off as much fat as you can. This should leave you with a lean and protein rich meal.

This is a chart of the leanest cuts of meat, with their calorie counts and fat and protein tallies. Use it to help you make wise meat choices.

3-OZ CUT	CALORIES	FAT (g)	PROTEIN (g)
BEEF			
Chuck shoulder	196	9	28
Eye round	156	6	25
Top round steak	162	5	27
Sirloin tip	162	6	24
Ground beef, extra lean	153	11	18
Sirloin steak	177	7	26
Filet mignon	174	8	24
Flank steak	207	13	22
PORK			
Center loin, chop	196	9	27
Fresh ham (picnic shoulder)	194	11	23
LAMB			
Leg	162	7	24
Loin chop	183	9	26
Shank	154	6	22
VEAL			
Cutlet	156	4	28
Shoulder steak	169	4	30
Chop	191	7	28

I.D. I.Q.

In the group below, identify which are highest in sugar.

A. Corn flakes   B. Frosted flakes   C. Shredded wheat   D. Raisin bran

Most cereals on the market today have a generous sprinkling of sugar. To find out which ones don't, look for specific labels ("No sugar added") or read the label yourself (we tell you how on page 89). Here, the cereal that is highest in sugar is frosted flakes; raisin bran is a close second. Plain corn flakes have about half the sugar of frosted, and shredded wheat has even less than that.

I.D. I.Q.

Identify which are the best fiber sources in the group below.

A. Applesauce   B. Potato chips   C. Biscuits   D. Grapes

In their original forms, apples, potatoes, and wheat for the biscuits are all fibrous. But the more they're cooked and processed, the more the fiber is broken down. For this reason, the grapes are the best fiber source.

In this fast-paced world, it's easy to rely on less-than-nutritious foods because they're convenient. But, something better could be just around the corner—the fruit stand.

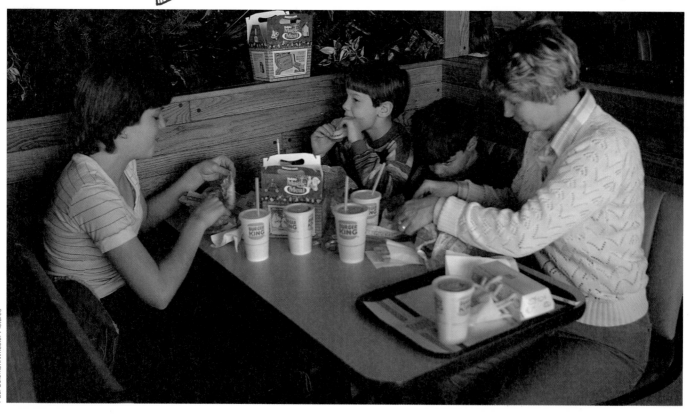

Paul Solomon/Wheeler Pictures

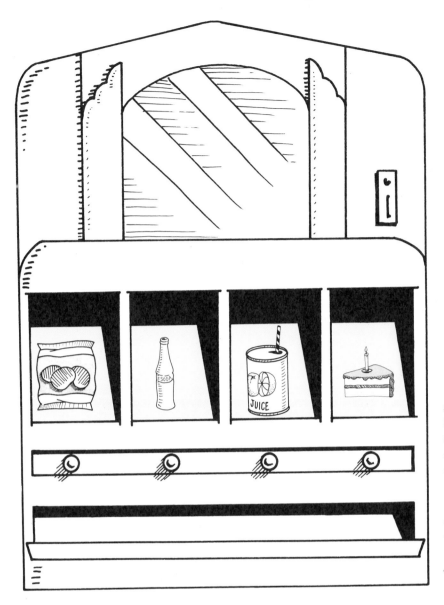

Snack time! Which would you choose? The selections from a vending machine or a concession stand are often limited to sugary pastries or salty and greasy potato chips. Better choices are whole-wheat crackers, frozen low-fat yogurt, or fruit juice.

HABIT TEST

It's not only what you eat, but *how* you eat it that matters. Watch out for these bad habits that sabotage good nutrition. How many of them are things you do regularly?

Because I'm so busy, I usually have to eat from a concession stand or a vending machine.

I eat my food very fast; it takes me less than fifteen minutes.

After I eat one plate of food, I go for seconds.

I can eat a whole jar of peanuts without even realizing it.

Even when I'm not hungry, I can't pass up food when others are eating.

I don't know what I'm going to eat until I see it.

I have a snack whenever I watch TV.

When there's nothing to do, my friends (or family) just go out for a bite.

True or False?

Fat should be cut off meat after you cook it.

False. If you can, trim all visible fat *before* you cook. This way, fat doesn't have a chance to cook back into the meat.

True or False?

Choose meat labeled ''prime'' at the supermarket.

False. Believe it or not, "prime" meats have the most fat. The United States Department of Agriculture grades meat on how tender it is, and fat makes meat more tender. Less fatty meats are labeled "choice" or "good."

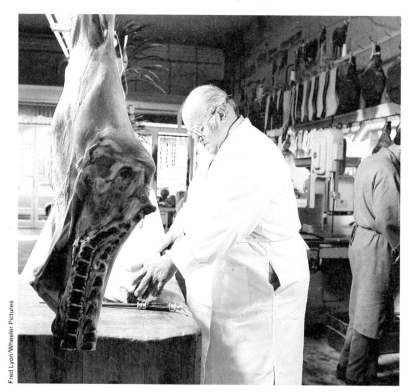

Fred Lyon/Wheeler Pictures

Because beef, pork, lamb, and veal can be high in fat, some people exclude them from their diets. However, lean red meat is an excellent source of protein and iron. The compromise is to eat them two or three times a week only.

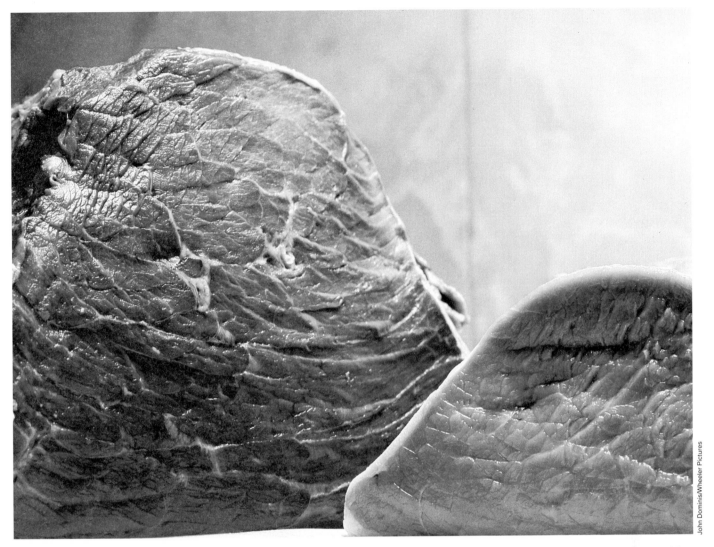

John Dominis/Wheeler Pictures

Red meat is made up of lean and fat. Lean is red; fat is white. Some fat is mixed in with the lean, and you can't do anything about it. But always trim off the fat from the outside edges of steak and chops.

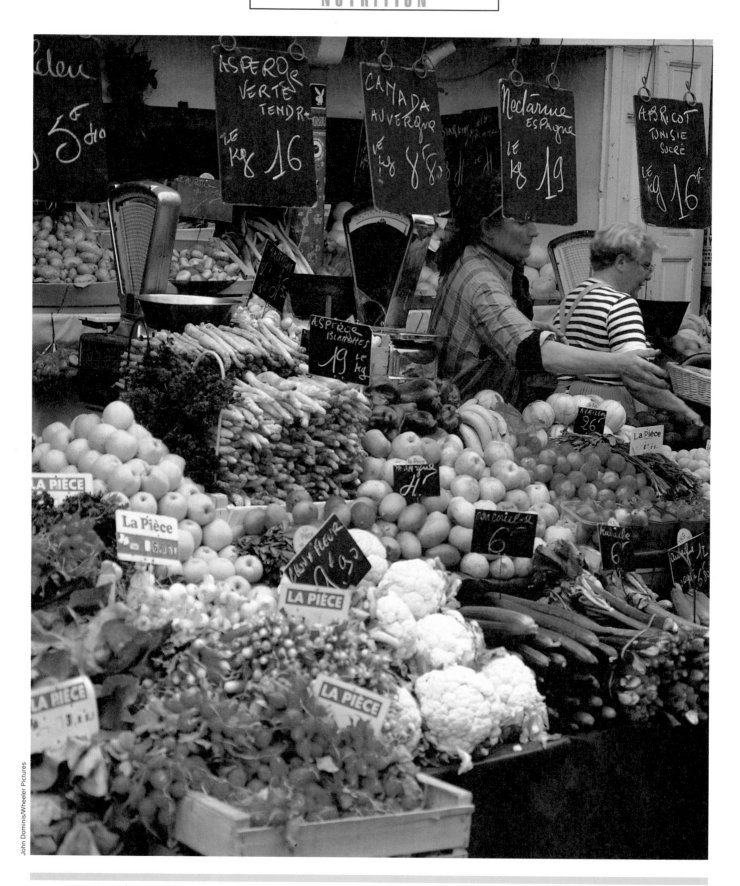

True or False?

Select foods labeled ''light'' or ''lite''; they're lower in fat.

False. Many times manufacturers use "light" to mean that a food *tastes* lighter or *weighs* less. The best way to tell if a product is low fat is to read the label. (We tell you how on page 89.)

True or False?

Use more egg whites than egg yolks.

True. Egg yolks have all the fat and cholesterol; whites are nearly pure protein. Try to make your omelets with one yolk and two whites.

Research shows that nearly 3,000 chemicals are added to foods during processing. You can't avoid all packaged foods, but be sure to eat more fresh fruits and vegetables.

What Can I Do To Improve My Nutrition?

I n Part I you read the basics about what effect good and bad nutrition can have on you. Now you must learn to apply this information and guidelines to your own life.

On the following pages, you'll take what you've learned so far and figure out how to use it. And *here's* where the need for everyone—particularly young people—to understand nutrition will be strongly emphasized. You need to have a clear idea of what a healthy diet *is* before you can eat one. Plus, you need some everyday food-choice advice for real-life situations. Between the many activities that you participate in each day, it isn't easy to juggle your calcium levels as well. Guidelines for making this easier are given here. You're already ahead of the game by showing an awareness and interest. Read on for some hands-on help.

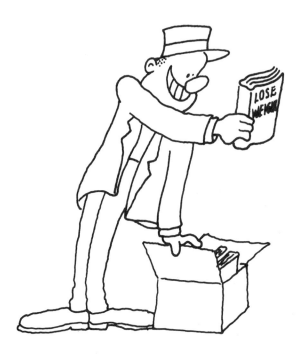

Know what makes a healthy diet.

Everybody wants to tell you how to eat: so-called diet experts who want to sell you their books; fast-food restaurants that want your business; scientists who truly believe their new research is the last word; even magazine and newspaper editors, who are sometimes too quick to write what they hear. With all this advice, recognizing a healthy diet is sometimes easier said than done.

That's the bad news. The good news is that by the time you finish reading this book, you'll be informed enough to figure out on your own if these people are sensible. You'll understand the USRDA's, your dietary guidelines, the four food groups, and some "ideal percentages." They sound complicated, but you'll see that all of them get at the same thing: a plan for a well-rounded diet. You don't have to memorize them, but it helps to be familiar with them. This way you can spot a suspicious nutrition claim as well as recognize a bad spot in your own diet.

USRDA's

USRDA's are United States Recommended Daily Allowances. They represent the government's most recent and best advice for how much of each essential nutrient you need—right down to the milligram. You'll often see them on food labels or hear them in commercials: "Contains 80 percent of the USRDA of iron."

It wouldn't help you much to give you all the RDA numbers, because in the first place they're too hard to remember. Also, it's not essential for you to get 100 percent of the USRDA of each nutrient every day. Why? The government makes them a little high so *everybody's* needs are satisfied (some people, like pregnant women, need more nutrients). What's more, government nutritionists figure that what you don't get in vitamin D one day, you'll get on another.

Some of the USRDA levels are more important than others. Use the following sections to find out if you're getting enough protein and calcium.

Sodium Check

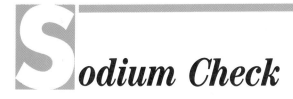

Write down all the salty foods that you've eaten in the past three days. Better yet, list all the foods you've eaten, then check the sodium content for each on the list below or the charts in the back of this book (pages 106–115). You'll be surprised to find that many foods you don't think of as salty actually contain a great deal of sodium. Total your sodium intake for all foods and divide that total by three.

Table salt, 1 teaspoon (5 grams): 2,000 milligrams
Bacon, 4 strips: 300 milligrams
Ham, 3 ounces (75 grams): 750 milligrams
Whole milk, 1 cup (235 milliliters): 120 milligrams
Cheddar cheese, 1 ounce (25 grams): 300 milligrams
Cottage cheese, 1 cup (200 grams): 450 milligrams
Butter, 1 tablespoon (⅔ British tablespoon): 150 milligrams
Prepared cereal, 1 cup (200 grams): 250 milligrams
Dill pickle, 1 large: 1,800 milligrams
Chicken noodle soup, 1 cup (235 milliliters): 975 milligrams
Tomato juice, 1 cup (235 milliliters): 500 milligrams
Catsup, 3 tablespoons (2 British Tablespoons): 500 milligrams
Soy sauce, 2 tablespoons (1⅓ British tablespoons): 2,500 milligrams
Potato chips, 8 ounces (200 grams): 2,250 milligrams
Baked Potato, 1 large: 6 milligrams
Ice cream, 1 cup (200 grams): 120 milligrams
Yogurt, 1 cup (200 grams): 160 milligrams
Chocolate chip cookie, 1 medium: 35 milligrams
Green beans, 1 cup (200 grams) fresh: 5 milligrams
Green beans, 1 cup (200 grams) canned: 320 milligrams

Your body only needs 200 milligrams of sodium each day, though 1,000 to 3,000 milligrams is considered "safe." Notice, however, that this is only about one-and-a-half teaspoons: Most of us consume much more than that. Even if you learn not to add table salt to everything—a bad habit many people need to break—most of the foods we eat are loaded with sodium. Your total sodium intake is probably much higher than it should be. Learn which are the high sodium foods, and avoid them. Choose low sodium alternatives, like a baked potato instead of potato chips (but don't load it up with butter and sour cream). After a while you won't even miss the salt.

Protein Check

Write down all the protein-rich foods you've eaten for the last three days. Find their values in the list below, then add them up and divide by three.

Bacon, 2 slices: 3.8 grams
*Beans, 1 cup (225 grams), cooked: 22 grams
Cheddar cheese, 1 ounce (25 grams): 7 grams
Cheese pizza, 2 slices: 15.6 grams
Chuck roast, 4 ounces (100 grams): 20 grams
Egg, 1 large: 7 grams
Ham, 1 4-ounce (100-gram) slice: 16.7 grams
Hamburger, 1 large: 26 grams
Hot dog, 1: 7 grams
*Low-fat yogurt, 1 cup: 11.9 grams
Pork chop, one small: 15.3 grams
Pork sausage, 2 links: 5 grams
*Skim milk, one cup: (235 milliliters): 9 grams
Tuna, one-half cup (115 grams), canned in oil: 23 grams
*Tuna, one-half cup (115 grams), canned in water: 28 grams
*Turkey, three ounces (75 grams): 27 grams

How many grams per day did you come up with? Girls from age eleven to eighteen need 46 grams; boys from eleven to fourteen need 45; and boys from fifteen to eighteen need 56. If you're like most people, you eat more than that. (Keep in mind that many other foods we didn't even mention have some protein, too.) At least you know you're getting all you need. But because foods high in protein are usually high in fat too, nutritionists tell us to cut back on protein—especially if you're over these numbers. For this reason, it's important to concentrate on the healthier choices, marked with an asterisk (*). Meat isn't the only source of protein, however. There are numerous other foods to choose from.

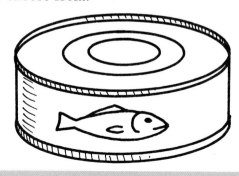

Calcium Check

Whereas protein is easy to overdo, calcium is hard to get enough of.

Write down all the calcium-rich foods you've eaten for the last three days. Find their values in the list below, then add them up and divide by three.

*Broccoli, 1 large stalk: 200 milligrams
*Canned salmon, one-half cup (115 grams): 250 milligrams
*Canned shrimp, one-half cup (115 grams): 150 milligrams
 Cheeseburger: 150 milligrams
 Cheese pizza, 2 slices: 350 milligrams
 Grated parmesan cheese, 2 tablespoons (1⅓ British tablespoons): 150 milligrams
 Ice cream, 1 cup (235 milliliters): 160 milligrams
*Ice milk, 1 cup (235 milliliters): 150 milligrams
 Instant cocoa, 1 cup (235 milliliters): 100 milligrams
*Low-fat cottage cheese, one-half cup (115 grams): 75 milligrams
*Low-fat yogurt, 1 cup (235 milliliters): 275 milligrams
*Sardines, 3 ounces (75 grams): 370 milligrams
*Skim milk, 1 cup (235 milliliters): 300 milligrams
*Spinach, one-half cup (100 grams), cooked: 115 milligrams
 Swiss cheese, 1 ounce (25 grams): 270 milligrams
*Tofu, 3½ ounces (48 grams): 125 milligrams
*Turnip greens, one-half cup (100 grams), cooked: 125 milligrams

Determine the amount of calcium you have consumed. Until you reach age nineteen, you'll need around 1,200 milligrams. (After that, male requirements drop to 800; female to 800 to 1,000.) As a rule of thumb, have four (one liter) cups of skim or low-fat milk and/or yogurt per day, and you'll get pretty much what you need. Because some calcium-rich foods are also high in fat, it's smart to depend on the low-fat foods, marked here with an asterisk (*). (see "Calcium for the Bones," page 18.)

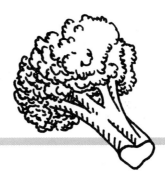

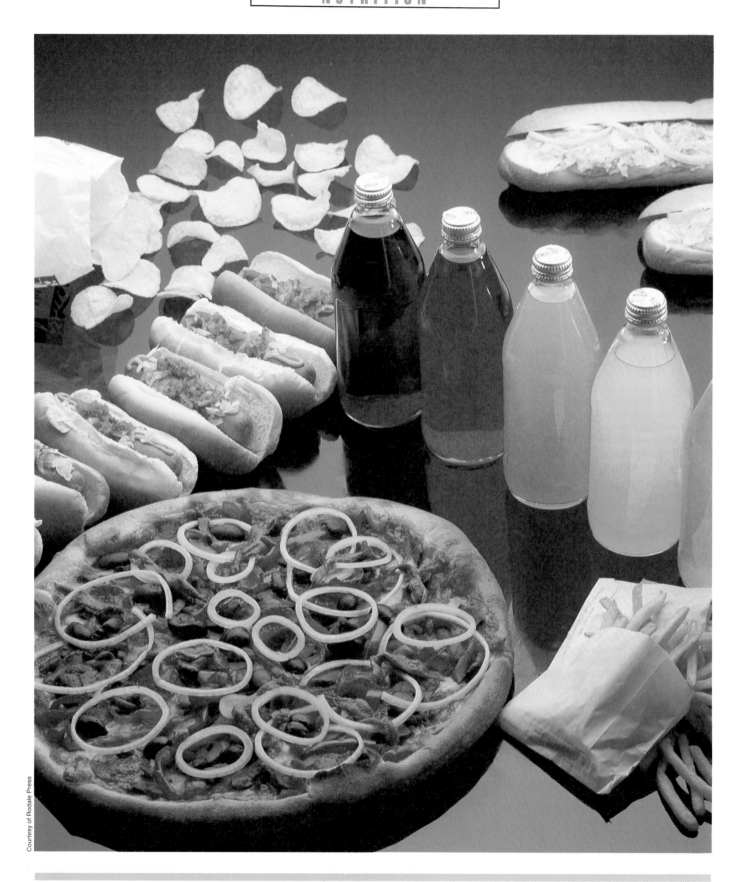

Dietary Guidelines

An easier plan to follow is the Dietary Guidelines for Americans, as provided by the United States Department of Agriculture and the United States Department of Health and Human Services. Instead of a list of numbers, these guidelines give you concrete, common-sense pointers. Let's look at those that apply to teenagers.

1. Eat a variety of foods.

The greater the variety, the less likely you are to have a shortage of an important nutrient. As you know, foods contain more than one nutrient, but no single food supplies everything you need.

2. Maintain an ideal weight.

By keeping your weight where it should be, you don't have to count every calorie. Without having to restrict many foods, you can have everything in moderation. Besides, obesity causes numerous health problems.

3. Avoid too much fat—especially saturated fat—and cholesterol.

This is a very important point. Although it's impossible to avoid all fat and cholesterol, concentrate on eating low-fat foods.

4. Eat foods with adequate starch and fiber.

Complex carbohydrates are excellent sources for these important dietary elements. They contain scores of nutrients and plenty of bulk, which aids digestion—often for fewer calories.

5. Avoid too much sugar.

We know that foods with calories *and* nutrients are better for us, but sugar is mostly calories. Sugar seems to cause fewer health problems than fat, but an excess can lead to obesity. An easy way to stay in shape, then, is to cut down on sugar.

6. Avoid too much sodium.

Although everyone needs some sodium, and people who have high blood pressure are more susceptible to sodium's risks, it is suspected that sodium-heavy diets can contribute to high blood pressure. In case you develop that problem someday, it certainly doesn't hurt to get into a good low-sodium habit now.

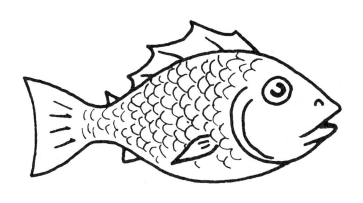

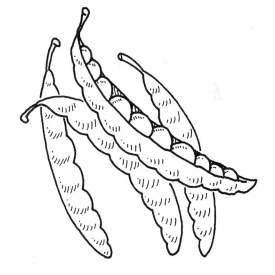

Face up to reality: At the mall, the school cafeteria, and maybe even at home, you could be tempted by high-fat, low-nutrient foods like these. However, many food businesses realize you want more nutritious choices and they are improving their menus. Speed up the process by passing along your personal preferences.

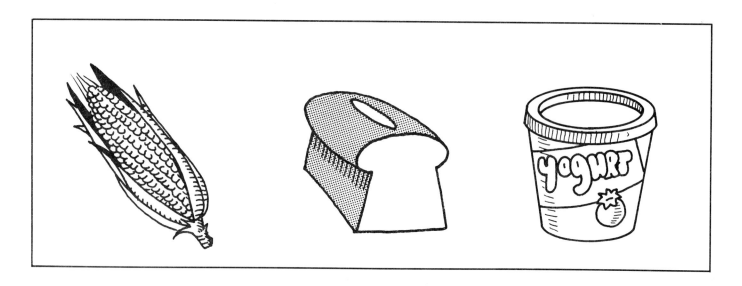

Food Groups

The four food groups are something you've heard about since you started school. Generally, these United States Department of Agriculture guidelines say teenagers need:

Three to four daily servings from the Milk Group
Low-fat milk, yogurt, cheese, ice milk, etc.
Two daily servings from the Meat (or Protein) Group
Poultry, fish, dry beans and peas, lean meat, etc.
Four daily servings from the Vegetable and Fruit Group
Four daily servings from the Bread and Cereal Group
Cooked and dried cereal, pasta, rice, bread.

These are good guidelines to keep in mind, given the following considerations:

#1. The Milk Group and Meat Group might also be called "The Fat Groups." You need all the calcium, protein, and vitamin D the Milk Group offers, and all the vitamins and protein the Meat Group offers. But you don't need all their fat. How do you get around it? Choose low-fat foods from both these groups—skim milk, low-fat yogurt and cheeses, ice milk instead of ice cream. In the Meat Group, concentrate on fish and poultry without skin. And when you eat red meats, select the leanest you can find. (See "The Difference Between Fat on Your Stomach and Fat on Your Plate," page 17).

#2. Vegetables and fruits are always a good dietary choice. Concentrate on unprocessed, fresh varieties for the best nutrition. Example: A baked potato has more fiber and less fat than scalloped potatoes. Be sure to include a good Vitamin-C source in your Fruit and Vegetable Group, such as deep yellow fruits (oranges, melons) or deep green vegetables (spinach, broccoli).

#3. You can have a sugary cereal four times a day and still not satisfy your Bread and Cereal Group requirement. The increased amount of sugar replaces the cereal with a lot of empty calories. Choose whole-grain or enriched cereals only—the less processed, the better.

Ideal Percentages

Finally, some nutritionists think it's better to talk in terms of "ideal percentages." Nutritionists recommend that protein make up about 10 to 15 percent of your daily calories; fats no more than 30 percent (preferably 10 to 20 percent); and carbohydrates 55 to 70 percent.

How do you fit this into your day? Take this into consideration: If you eat like the typical person, you get 60 percent of your calories from fat and added sugars. That means you must get about 40 percent of your calories from proteins and carbohydrates *combined*. So you need to cut out about half of the fat- and sugar-heavy foods you eat, which include not only junk foods like potato chips and candy bars, but also high-fat meats and dairy foods.

When it comes to protein, even if you're eating the recommended 15 percent (and statistics say you're probably getting more), that leaves you only 25 percent for complex carbohydrates. By reducing your fats, you'll probably automatically lower the protein if it's already over the recommended 15 percent. Go full speed ahead with the complex carbohydrates by doubling or even tripling what you've been eating.

Recommended Daily Percentages
10–15% Proteins
10–30% Fats
55–70% Complex carbohydrates

Average American Diet
60% Fats and added sugars
40% Proteins and complex carbohydrates

Solution
(1) Cut fats and added sugars in half.
(2) Double complex carbohydrate intake.

At the top of the "good-for-you" food list are green vegetables. Not only are they typically rich in vitamin A and C, many—like peas, broccoli, and cabbage—are high in fiber. That means that green veggies help fight disease as they fortify you.

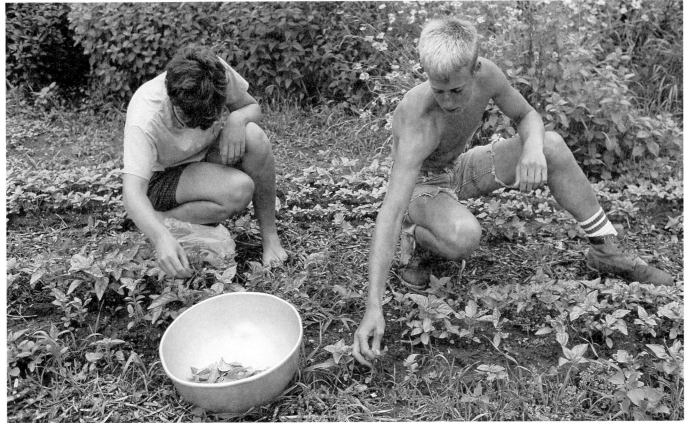

Susan Lapides/Wheeler Pictures

Special Needs, Special Diets

So far, we've talked about the basic diet requirements for healthy people, but needs do vary. For example, diabetics should limit foods heavy in sugar and fat as a matter of life and death. Pregnant or breastfeeding women have to boost their calories and nutrients. Sick people must follow prescribed diets based on their needs.

Because special diets need the sure hand of a doctor, we're not going to outline any here. Some of you, however, might actually need a little more or a little less of some of the basic requirements we've described.

Weight-loss diets also depend on individual needs. Although they're taken a little too casually by many people, they've no doubt saved a few lives. We know that 40 percent of the population—two in every five people—is overweight by twenty pounds (seven and a half kilos) or more. A successful weight-loss program would lower the risk of disease.

Yet there's a difference between a healthy weight-loss diet and an unhealthy one. Too many people rely on special blender drinks or reducing drugs instead of good, old-fashioned, simple eating. And then, because they lose the weight too fast and don't change their eating habits on the way, those people gain the weight right back. Gaining and losing weight over and over again—the "yo-yo syndrome"—has been shown to be unhealthy. What's more, it makes losing weight harder every time.

By eating a variety of foods, cutting back on fats and sugars, and exercising regularly, overweight people can lose weight healthfully and keep it off. Of course, this is the basic health prescription for everyone—a healthy diet is a way of life. By eating good foods all the time, you stay in shape and you feel good—all the time.

But what if you really do need a weight-loss plan? There are plenty of reasons why a teenager shouldn't diet (see box). See a doctor, and he or she will tell you if you need to lose and how. In the meantime, follow our pointers for "Loading Up, Cutting Back" on page 82, as well as "Weight-Loss Wisdom" on page 72.

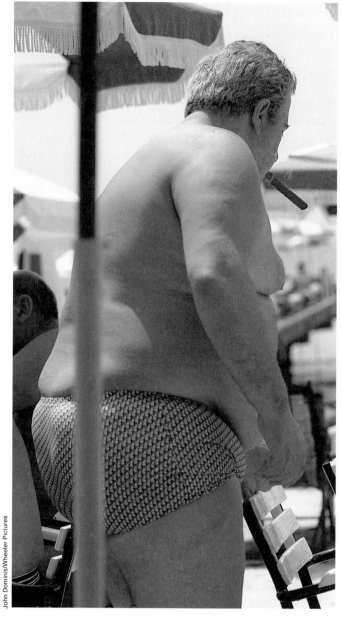

John Dominis/Wheeler Pictures

It's easy to see that extra weight is unattractive, but besides that, it's very unhealthy. Obese people are at higher risk of heart disease, diabetes, and many other problems.

Good Reasons Not to Try to Lose Weight

1. Growing bodies need more calories than grown ones.

Hands down, this is the best reason for not putting yourself on a minimum-calorie diet. You've got enough going on inside of you right now—don't force your body to work on a shortage of nutrients.

2. Busy schedules and larger bodies need more calories.

If you're bouncing from choir practice to dance committee meetings to gym class, you need more calories to keep going. And if you're 5'8" (173 centimeters), you need more calories than your 5'1" (155-centimeter) friend. Now how can *you* be sure how many calories you need to accommodate your lifestyle? Ask the doctor to help you assess that.

3. You won't feel as energetic.

Let's clarify this statement a bit: If you're living on snack foods, you probably don't feel like exercising. But you're going to feel really bad—healthy diet or not—when you cut yourself down to nothing.

4. You'll feel like you're punishing yourself.

This is a problem for adult dieters, too. They feel deprived by cutting out all the foods they like, so one day they lose control and demolish the snack section at a local supermarket. Don't ever exclude *everything* you enjoy, but always eat in moderation. If you deny yourself, you could end up eating even more of the foods you're trying to avoid.

5. You'll have a negative outlook and an incomplete diet.

It wouldn't hurt most of us to eliminate some fatty and sugary foods. But if you're consuming only carrot sticks and grapefruit juice—you will eventually become bored and discouraged. Additionally, you will be malnourished. All sorts of foods are needed for a nutritious diet—not just one or two.

utrition Nuts: Beware!

Just because a diet book sells in the millions or a diet pill seems to have amazing results doesn't mean it is a sound solution to weight problems. It's not wise to try any of them. Here's what to look out for:

Diet Books

Whether the author is a doctor or not, it's not always easy to tell if he or she is qualified to tell you what to eat. Be especially careful of books that rely on one or two food groups or which eliminate many. For example, steer clear of a "Grapefruit Diet" or a "Popcorn Diet."

Testimonies

You'd be surprised what a person will say when he or she is paid enough money. It *could* be true that a person in an advertisement lost a substantial amount of weight by using a diet pill. However, the ad will not tell you whether the person also dieted or exercised to lose pounds, or whether the person damaged his or her health by taking the pills.

Supplements (drinks, pills, powders, etc.)

Real food is the key; chemicals from a laboratory will not help you lose weight in the long run.

Gadgets

Such items as rubber tubing worn around the waist do not really help you sweat off extra pounds. With these devices you don't lose pounds—you lose water. After drinking a couple of glasses of liquids, your waistline is back to normal.

Quick Cures

It's been proven time and time again that a good weight loss is accomplished carefully and slowly, at about one to two pounds (about a kilo) per week. Anybody who loses fifteen pounds (five and a half kilos) in 10 days didn't really lose fat; he lost body fluids, and the first time he goes back to normal eating he's going to gain it right back. Remember: Any promise of losing more than two pounds (a kilo) per week is quackery.

Anything else that looks too good to be true probably is.

When it comes to good nutrition, everyday events can knock you for a loop. For example, although popcorn can be a healthy snack, movie-theater popcorn is popped in fatty oil—not to mention drenched in ''butter'' and salt. Air-popped corn is better.

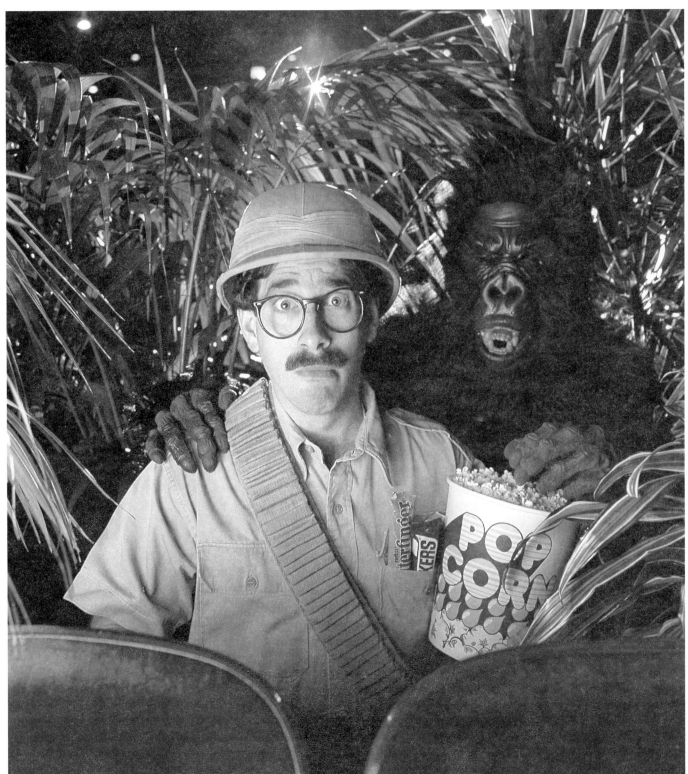

John Dominis/Wheeler Pictures

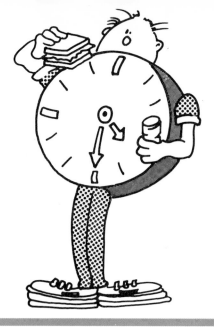

W eight-Loss Wisdom

A doctor will tell you that the best way to lose weight is to cut back on fats and sugars and to exercise. In addition, here are some easy, non-health-threatening tricks:

Stop eating by the clock. If you're not hungry when your mother brings out the after-school snacks at 4:30 then don't eat them.

Be aware of what you're eating. Be aware of what you put into your mouth and make an effort to truly taste each bite. In this way, you're bound to eat less.

Stop and think about why you're eating. Don't eat simply because you're in a situation in which you would normally eat. Only eat because you are hungry—not because you are depressed or bored.

Don't skip meals. Skipping meals may sound like a good diet idea, but it's not. For example, if you don't eat breakfast, you're going to be dying for more fattening foods at lunch.

Keep "bad foods" out of sight. If the coffee-table candy bowl stops you in your tracks every time, ask Mom or Dad to put it away, or replace the candy with some grapes. Sometimes it's not how much you eat, but what you eat that causes problems.

Don't eat fast. It takes a little while for the nerves in your stomach to signal a full feeling to your brain, slow down and you'll feel fuller faster. Try this: Put your fork down between bites; take smaller bites; taste each bite and enjoy it more!

Pre-load your meals. In other words, have something very early in your meal to fill you up more quickly. Research shows that people who eat soup before a full dinner actually eat less. Don't counteract your good intentions with a creamy, fattening soup, though. Instead, have some vegetable soup or something clearer—like a broth. (A light salad or glass of water might also do the trick).

Put less food on your plate. And remove your plate or get up from the table when you're finished.

Almost all diets tell you to drink at least eight glasses of water a day. The truth is that anyone, dieters and non-dieters, should drink that much and more. The two charts below will help you understand why. The chart on the bottom shows how your body uses all that H_2O, and the one on the top shows you where you can get water besides from the faucet.

WATER DOESN'T COME FROM THE FAUCET ALONE!

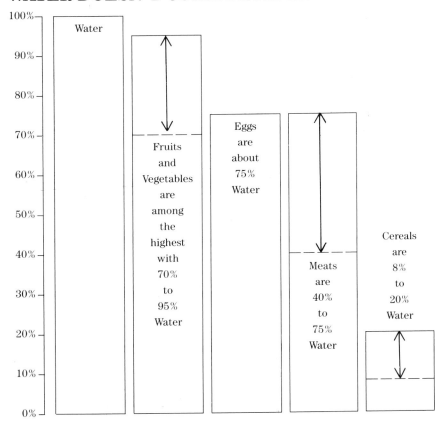

WHERE DOES THE WATER GO?

1 The body usually loses 2½ to 3 quarts of water every day (12 glasses).

2 The kidneys use about 5½ glasses of water every day.

3 The lungs take about 2 glasses of water every day.

4 The skin uses about 2 glasses of water every day.

5 Breathing takes about 1⅓ glasses of water every day.

6 The intestines use about ½ glass of water every day.

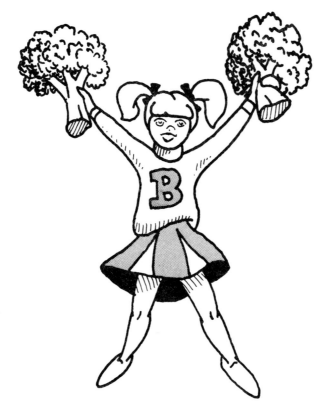

Are you underweight? Although many may envy your situation, you may be quite unhappy with the way you look. Once again, it's important to get the doctor's word to know if you actually are underweight, and, if so, what to do about it. It could be that illness is affecting your appetite.

But don't think for one minute that loading up on fatty foods will fill you out. They might, but they won't do it in a healthy way. Instead, try these pointers:

○ Eat at least three meals a day. If your appetite is small, eat several smaller meals.
○ It's okay to select higher-calorie foods, but make sure they're nutritious. Eat lots of whole-grain breads and low-fat dairy products.
○ Snack on healthy foods, but don't have them too close to dinner.
○ Make meal time as important as any other appointment on your schedule.

People who spend considerable time exercising also have special diet needs. Don't fall back on that old myth about protein being the mainstay of an athletic diet. True, it's important for building tissues, but protein doesn't build muscles. Exercise does. And an overload of fatty proteins will only serve to slow down muscle function and development.

What athletes *do* need is quick energy and staying power—both of which are provided by complex carbohydrates. That's not to say that you should eat only complex carbohydrates; like everyone else, athletes need a varied diet. Still, you'll probably find that nutrient- and fiber-dense foods will help your performance.

Athletes should also focus on water. If you're sweating, you're losing water. Don't wait until you are thirsty to drink water; by that time, your body needs water more than you realize. Be sure to drink water before and after a workout—at least six to eight glasses a day—and don't stop when you no longer feel thirsty.

As for salt pills and the thirst-quenching athletic drinks on the market, they simply don't measure up to more natural methods for salt replenishment. You'll get back the salt you lose through sweating by eating a good diet. Athletic drinks won't hurt you, but water is the best body-satisfier.

Especially for Women

If you've already begun to menstruate, you may have problems with cramps, weight gain, headaches, and other discomforts. This is because your hormones are playing games (it's natural), and while they help to regulate your period, they also hang on to the salt in your body, making you feel bloated. They keep your body from using sugar, so you crave something sweet; and produce substances that cause uterine cramps.

How can you help yourself with nutrition?

1. Cut back on salty foods for about two weeks before your period.
2. Drink lots of water to flush out excess salt.
3. Satisfy yourself with a sweet, but try to make it something healthy, like kiwifruit or a banana.
4. Eat iron-rich floods (beans, fish, poultry) to help replace the iron you lose in menstrual blood.

The Vegetarian Diet

People have different reasons for eating an all-vegetable diet. Some say they don't like to kill animals. Others don't want to eat the chemicals fed to animals to protect them from diseases. Still others concentrate on vegetables because they're so low in fat and cholesterol.

For some this diet works, but it's a tough balancing act. Some of the nutrients we typically get from meat (protein, iron, and vitamin B12) are not found in many vegetables. So vegetarians have to go to a lot of trouble to make sure they eat the vegetables that contain these nutrients. It is possible to eat a completely nutritious diet of only vegetables, but it's not easy. Sometimes vegetarians have to rely on supplements, which aren't as good as getting nutrients directly from food. For now it's probably best for you to concentrate on eating a well-balanced diet without having to worry about these problems.

Take charge!

Vitamins and nutrients have to be carefully balanced in your diet. In order to have the wholesome diet you want, you're going to have to choose, ask, and work for it. Here are the day-to-day basics to get you started.

Choices

Ultimately, of course, it comes down to making a choice. Are you going to have the hamburger and fries or the baked chicken and green beans? Is it going to be a chocolate-chip cookie or a piece of fruit?

That may be a tough decision, but it's one you're going to have to make several times a day. The calorie comparisons here will help you decide.

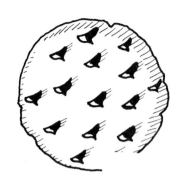

Everyday Disorders

There are several minor adjustments you can make in your diet for those little discomforts in life. For example:

Constipation:

Ideally you'll have a bowel movement anywhere from two to three times a day to once every two or three days. If you're having problems, a diet high in fiber and water will help. See a doctor if this is a common occurence.

Diarrhea:

This is the other side of constipation. Although it could be a symptom of any of several illnesses, it could also be triggered by something you ate. Look out for very spicy foods; lack of food variety; too much food; food that has been improperly cooked or handled; or too much caffeine.

Indigestion, heartburn, gas, or belching:

Try to cut out foods that usually give you problems. Pinpoint these foods, and avoid them in the future. If you have recurrent problems, see a doctor.

The calories in
1 BANANA SPLIT (3 SCOOPS OF ICE CREAM, 1 BANANA, HOT FUDGE, WHIPPED
CREAM, NUTS, AND MARASCHINO CHERRIES)
Are equal to the calories in
1 16-POUND (7-KILOGRAM) WATERMELON

or

21 AND A 1/2 CUPS (2 KILOGRAMS) OF CHERRIES

or

60 SWEET GHERKIN PICKLES

The calories in
1 8-OUNCE (225-GRAM) BAG OF ONION-AND-SOUR CREAM-FLAVORED POTATO
CHIPS
Are equal to the calories in
8 1/2 BAKED POTATOES, EACH WITH 2 TABLESPOONS (1⅓ BRITISH
TABLESPOONS) OF SOUR CREAM

or

11 BAKED POTATOES WITHOUT SOUR CREAM

or

47 GRAHAM CRACKERS

or

61 CARROTS

The calories in
1 LARGE FAST-FOOD HAMBURGER AND 1 SERVING OF FRENCH FRIES
Are equal to the calories in
1 3-POUND (1⅓-KILOGRAM) BROILED CHICKEN
(with skin trimmed)

or

9 8-OUNCE (235 MILLILITER) CANS OF TOMATO SOUP

or

56 MEDIUM OYSTERS

The calories in
A BREAKFAST OF 3 PANCAKES, BUTTER, AND SYRUP
Are equal to the calories in
9 BOWLS OF OATS

or

10 BOILED EGGS

or

11 APPLES

That's not even taking into consideration the overdose of sugar and fat you get in these high-calorie foods. Take a look at this:

1 GLASS OF WHOLE MILK
Has the same amount of fat as
20 GLASSES OF SKIM MILK

1 SERVING OF SAUSAGE
Has the same amount of fat as
4 ⅓ SERVINGS OF STEAMED SHRIMP

1 BROWNIE
Has the same amount of fat as
31 CUPS (5 KILOGRAMS) OF RAISINS

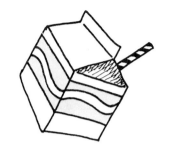

We could go on with these kinds of comparisons for pages. It's a matter of perspective, something you can sum up in your own head as you're weighing a decision between salted cashews or carrot sticks; macaroni and cheese or wild rice. You get more for your calories with healthier foods.

This formula should help you make the right choices: a gram of fat has nine calories, whereas a gram of complex carbohydrate has four. A gram of sugar has four calories, too. But since calories are often highly concentrated in sugar-sweetened foods, you can eat too much sugar before you're satisfied. Example: Compare three bananas with one two-ounce (fifty-gram) candy bar. Both have about the same carbohydrate content, but you're probably going to stop after eating one or two bananas. On the other hand, you'll probably eat the *whole* candy bar.

For more on sugar and fat comparisons, turn to page 82.

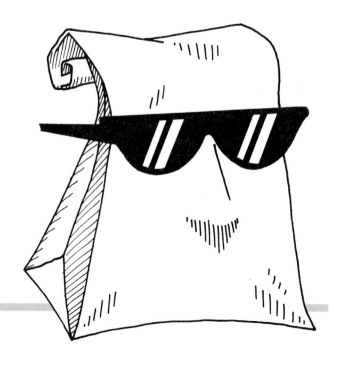

Is it ''cool'' at your school to bring your lunch, or does everyone eat in the cafeteria? In either case, make nutritious choices. Poor health from bad nutrition is definitely not ''cool.''

an You Find the Nutritional Mistake?

1. Monica knows that whole-wheat pancakes are good for her, so she made some for breakfast. With butter and syrup, she couldn't even tell the difference in the taste from regular pancakes.
2. Boiled eggs aren't cooked with oil like fried ones are, so Allen has two every morning.
3. Thelma has been drinking sodas that have added fruit juices ever since they first came out; she figures she'll get more vitamins from them.
4. Phil is trying to lose weight, so he eats frozen yogurt with fruit every day at lunch.
5. When Pat found out that spaghetti was healthy, she was thrilled. She eats it as often as she can, trying out different toppings: tomato sauces; butter and garlic; ground beef; and creamy cheese sauce.
6. At fast-food restaurants, Bill takes the bread off his hamburgers to save calories.
7. Elizabeth has her nutritional bases covered; she only buys foods with "natural" ingredients.
8. Here is Sarah's lunch: turkey, mozzarella, tomato, and mayonnaise on white bread.
9. Herman likes to alternate his protein choices. Since he had a high-fat pork chop for lunch, he'll have fried fish tonight.
10. At the party, Katie avoided the potato chips and filled up instead on cut vegetables, dip, cheese, and whole-wheat crackers.

Turn to the next page for the answers.

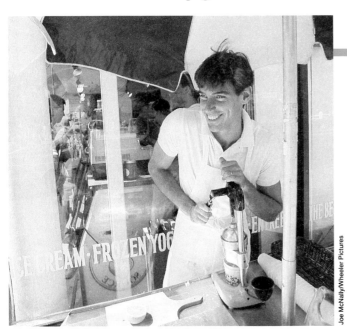

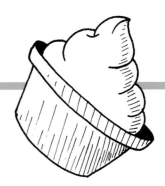

Joe McNally/Wheeler Pictures

Frozen desserts are tricky because some are good for you and some aren't. Check the ingredients and look for low-fat frozen yogurt, fruity sorbets, fruit bars, and ice milk. Steer clear of gourmet ice creams packed with fat and sugar.

nswers to *"Can You Find the Nutritional Mistake?"*

These are other examples of the daily choices you'll have to make during your search for a nutritionally sound diet. How did you do?

1. Monica did well to make whole-wheat pancakes, but she canceled out everything by smothering them in butter and syrup. Try sliced strawberries as a topper instead.

2. Allen's right: Boiled eggs are better than fried, scrambled, or omelets. However, nobody needs to eat two eggs a day. Three eggs per week is the recommendation.

3. Thelma is getting a bare-bones minimum of vitamins from fruit juices added to sodas. Unless she is drinking a diet soda, she's getting too much sugar. Fruit juice is a better choice.

4. If it's low-fat frozen yogurt, it's a good choice—especially with the fruit. Phil would be better off, however, by eating a variety of different foods instead of focusing on one. Beware: Frozen yogurts often have more sugar and fat than regular yogurts.

5. Pat has made a good choice in selecting the tomato sauces, but the rest of those toppings are filled with fat.

6. Plenty of people besides Bill don't realize that beef has much more fat than bread. You'd be better off leaving the *hamburger* off. Or instead of ordering one of those burgers with two quarter-pound (100-gram) patties, order one small burger instead—even two small burgers are better than a big one. Best bet of all, order broiled chicken (when it's available) or lean roast beef. The high-fat content of fried foods makes most fast foods unhealthy.

7. Elizabeth doesn't know that sugar is natural. The natural food companies can *bathe* your food in sugar or honey and call it "natural." (see "Health Foods: Not Always What They Seem," page 92).

8. Sarah is a smart girl. The turkey and tomato are grade-A choices, but she would have done even better to make the bread whole-wheat, leave off or specify low-fat cheese (low-fat mozzarella is often "part-skim," meaning it was made with skim milk instead of whole milk), and substituting mustard for mayo.

9. Herman might as well have pork chops for supper every night. Deep-fry the fish in oil, and you're adding greasy fat to your diet. Broiled, grilled, or baked fish or pork chops are better choices.

10. It was wise of Katie to avoid the potato chips. But if the dip was made with sour cream, it should be avoided. Then there's the cheese and crackers. The whole-wheat crackers are pretty good fare at a party, but watch out for that cheese: It has a high fat content. Softer cheeses—goat, farmer—are generally lower in fat than hard cheeses. Skip all processed cheeses (they're usually marketed as individually wrapped "sandwich slices," or they're whipped and packaged in a jar or canister); they're high in fat, low in natural nutrients.

Hard cheeses, such as Parmesan, cheddar or Swiss, are high in fat. Opt for low-fat soft cheeses such as low-fat cottage cheese, part-skim mozzarella, or part-skim ricotta.

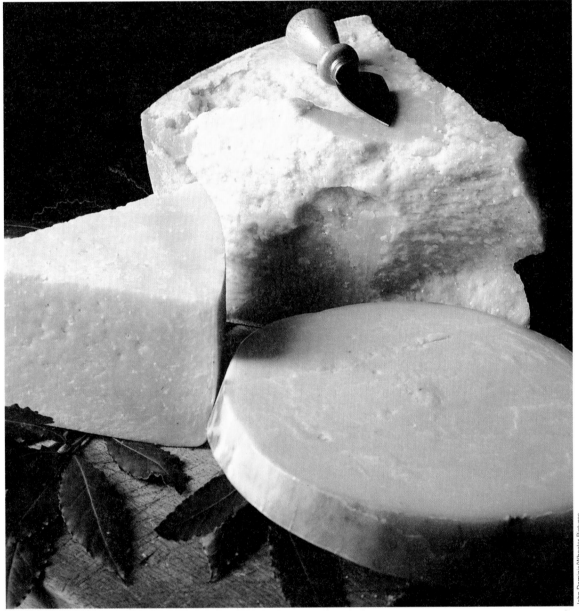

John Dominis/Wheeler Pictures

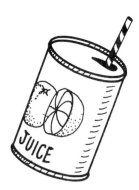

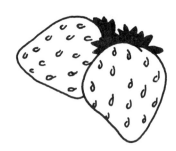

Loading Up, Cutting Back

We've discussed adding, cutting, avoiding, and substituting good foods for bad foods, and you will find numerous helpful suggestions throughout this book. But if you want a good, solid list of ways to work different food into/out of your diet, you should follow these rules:

For Less Fat:

○ Cut away any fat you can see on your meat.
○ Pull the skin off chicken and turkey.
○ Spray pans with no-stick spray instead of coating them with oil or butter. Try to minimize all the butter, margarine, and oil you use in any cooking.
○ Use low-cholesterol fats for cooking, such as safflower and olive oil.
○ Don't butter your bread.
○ Use more egg whites than egg yolks in your dishes.
○ Choose lean cuts of meats: flank steak, sirloin tip, London broil, boiled ham, leg of lamb, veal.
○ Eat more fish. Fish has fat, but its fat is healthier than red-meat fat.
○ Rely on low-fat dairy products: ice milk, low-fat yogurt, skim milk, ricotta cheese, part-skim cheeses.
○ Substitute English muffins, bagels, or pita bread (preferably whole-wheat) for fat-rich biscuits, croissants, and muffins.

○ Watch out for creamy soups; clearer ones are usually lower in fat.
○ Use more vinegar, less oil on your salads; avoid creamy, mayonnaise-based dressings.
○ Eat more fresh and raw foods; less packaged, processed, or cooked foods.
○ Buy tuna "packed in water" instead of tuna "packed in vegetable oil."
○ Steam, grill, stir-fry, roast, boil, stew, broil or bake meats, poultry, and fish on a rack; sauté in a little oil, or poach in water for lower-fat cooking.

For Less Sugar:

○ Never add sugar to your food.
○ Substitute fresh fruit for desserts.
○ Drink fruit juices and water instead of soda.
○ Season foods with spices (cinnamon, cardamom, ginger, cloves, allspice, almond, vanilla, peppermint) instead of sugar.
○ Eat less packaged, processed foods, more fresh and raw foods.
○ Choose cereals that aren't pre-sweetened.
○ Watch out for condiments, like ketchup and French dressing; they have loads of "hidden sugars."
○ Buy fruit "packed in its own juice" instead of those "in heavy syrup."
○ Beware of gum, cough drops, mints, candies.
○ Look for "100 percent pure, no sugar added" fruit juices.

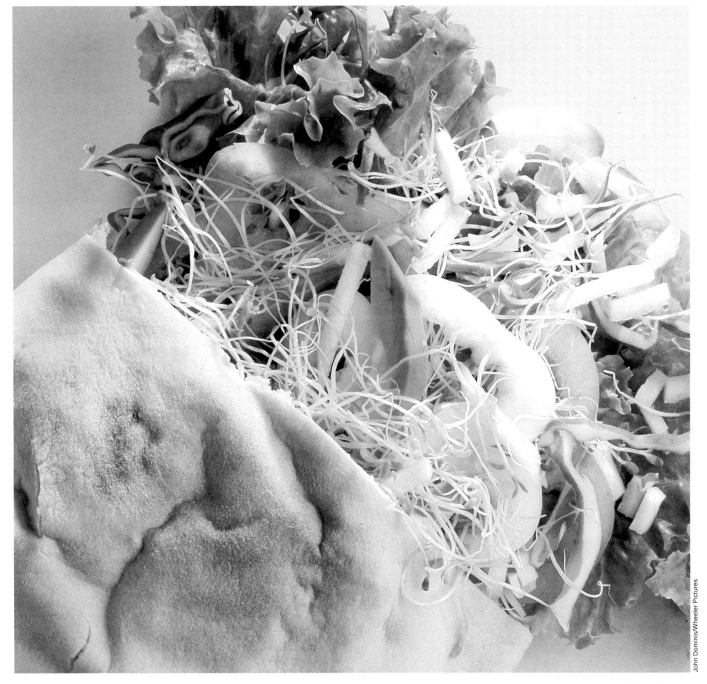

John Dominis/Wheeler Pictures

Instead of fatty cheeses, lunch meats, and mayonnaise, stuff your sandwich with vegetables and a vinegary dressing or mustard.

For More Fiber:

○ Choose whole-grain foods when you can: whole-wheat instead of white bread; bran muffins instead of blueberry; rolled oats instead of pre-sweetened cereals.
○ Eat foods raw instead of cooked; cooking breaks down fiber.
○ Have cooked, dried beans and peas instead of canned.
○ Eat fruits such as apples and vegetables such as potatoes with their skins.
○ Snack on unbuttered popcorn.
○ Substitute fruits for fruit juices.
○ Add salads to your meals. Fortify them with shredded carrots and cabbage, cauliflower, apple slices, beets, or beans.
○ Choose soups with brown rice, barley, vegetables, or beans.
○ Add green peppers, celery, or tomatoes to pasta sauces.
○ Put crunchy vegetables in your sandwiches: lettuce, carrots, bean sprouts, cucumbers.
○ Mix raisins, pineapples, peaches, or cantaloupe into low-fat yogurt or cottage cheese.
○ Substitute whole-wheat flour for white when baking.
○ Read the labels on boxes of so-called high-fiber cereals for their exact contents. Choose the one with the most dietary fiber, the least sugar. (Find out more about food labels on page 89.)

○ Add fiber to your diet gradually and drink lots of water.

For More Calcium:

○ Melt low-fat cheeses over vegetables or sandwiches.
○ Make milk shakes with skim milk, fruit, and ice in a blender.
○ Make salad dressings with low-fat yogurt.
○ Use skim milk instead of water to make hot cereals.
○ Slip some tofu into your salads or other dishes.
○ Toss salads with low-fat cheese.
○ Snack on low-fat cottage cheese or yogurt.
○ Boost your diet with green, leafy vegetables: spinach, collard greens, and turnip greens.
○ Eat more canned fish, which includes calcium-rich fish bones: salmon, tuna, and sardines.
○ Watch for new calcium-enriched foods on the market: milks, cereals, flours, even sugar-free hot chocolate mixes.

For More Water:

○ Drink at least six to eight glasses of water a day.
○ Drink even when you're not thirsty.
○ Eat lots of fresh vegetables and fruits, which also contain water.
○ Try sparkling waters and mineral waters instead of soda.
○ Stop by every water fountain for a sip.

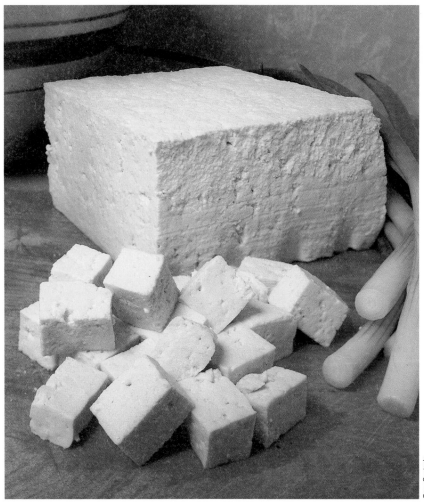

Tony Cenicola

 What is tofu?

A. Tofu is a white, nearly tasteless blend of soybeans and water from Asia. It usually comes in a dense, congealed square and is a bit smoother and chewier than ricotta. Nutritionists consider it to be one of our nearly perfect foods. Not only is it very low in calories, it's cholesterol-free and high in protein, calcium, B vitamins, and iron. *And* it's inexpensive!

Although tofu has very little taste of its own, it has the remarkable ability to "adopt" the taste of other foods it's combined with. For example, tofu mixed in lasagna may have a different texture, but it basically tastes like the tomato sauce, cheese, and seasonings it accompanies. This ancient food form also makes a good substitute for eggs, creams, and cheese; low-calorie test kitchens often use tofu in cheesecakes, pies, milk shakes, and pizzas. Toss a few chunks in soups, salads, and casseroles to boost the nutritional content without boosting fat or calories.

Fiber Guide

The National Cancer Institute recommends that you take in between 20 and 35 grams of fiber daily. Follow your intake for a few days to see what you average. Then read how to add more fiber to your diet on page 84.

Cereals

Extra-fiber bran (1 ounce) . . . . .13 grams
Bran (1 ounce). . . . . .9 grams
Raisin bran (1 ounce) . . . . .4 grams
Hot oats (1 ounce). . . . . .2 grams

Greens and beans

Baked beans with tomato sauce (½ cup, cooked). . . . . .9 grams
Kidney beans (½ cup, cooked) . . . . .7 grams
Lima and pinto beans (½ cup, cooked) . . . . .5 grams
Peas (½ cup, cooked). . . . . .4 grams
Corn (canned) (½ cup, cooked) . . . . .3 grams
Potato with skin, sweet potato with skin (½ of a large potato) . . . . .3 grams
Broccoli, brussels sprouts (½ cup, cooked). . . . . .2 grams
Carrots, spinach, zucchini (½ cup, cooked) . . . . .2 grams

Breads and pastas

Whole-wheat spaghetti, cooked (1 cup) . . . . .4 grams
Bran muffin (1 medium). . . . . .3 grams
Whole-wheat bread (2 slices) . . . . .3 grams
Whole-wheat English muffin (1 slice) . . . . .3 grams
Whole-wheat pancakes (2) . . . . .3 grams
Brown rice (½ cup or 100 grams, cooked) . . . . .1 gram

Fruits

Blackberries (½ cup or 100 grams) . . . . .5 grams
Pear with skin . . . . .5 grams
Apple with skin. . . . . .4 grams
Prunes (4). . . . . .4 grams
Orange . . . . .3 grams
Raisins (¼ cup or 50 grams) . . . . .3 grams
Strawberries (1 cup or 100 grams). . . . . .3 grams
Banana. . . . . .2 grams
Peach with skin. . . . . .2 grams
Blueberries (½ cup or 50 grams) . . . . .2 grams
Pineapple (1 cup or 100 grams) . . . . .2 grams

Miscellaneous

Bran crackers (1 cracker) . . . . .3 grams
Wheat germ (3 tablespoons or 2 British tablespoons) . . . . .3 grams
Crispbreads (2 crackers) . . . . .2 grams
Popcorn (3 cups unbuttered, or 2.5 ounces/63 milligrams, unpopped). . . . . .2 grams
Celery (3 stalks). . . . . .2 grams
Whole-wheat oatmeal cookies with raisins (3) . . . . .2 grams

Shopping Savvy

Maybe you're used to running through the super-market without giving thought to the nutritional content of what you're purchasing.

After reading this section you will see the local grocery store with new eyes. It's a wealth of information and full of consumer traps.

Things to know:

○ Fresh foods are cheaper than packaged foods.
○ Candies are placed at the checkout line with hopes that you'll make a last-minute choice.
○ You'll buy more food if you shop when you're hungry.
○ You have to root out the healthy choices yourself; food labels don't always mean what they

seem to say, even though the Food and Drug Administration oversees them.

Meats labeled *prime* have the most fat. Less fatty meats are labeled *choice, good,* or better yet, *lean* and *extra lean.*

A company can call meat *lite, leaner,* or *lower fat* if the product has 25 percent less fat or cholesterol compared to USDA standards for that meat product. If the meat is labeled *lean* or *lowfat,* it has 10 percent less fat and cholesterol. Foods labeled *lite* or *light* aren't necessarily lower in calories. These terms could mean the food is lighter in weight and texture.

Reduced calorie means a product has one-third fewer calories than it would normally have (the manufacturers have cut out some fattening ingredients).

Low-calorie means a product has no more than forty calories per serving.

There are no official definitions of *natural.*

When certain nutrients are lost in foods during refining and processing, manufacturers sometimes add some of them back. They are then labeled *enriched.*

Fortified foods have nutrients added beyond the natural levels.

As you can see, many of these labels are confusing. A "reduced-calorie" food might actually contain more calories than a food naturally low in calories. A "natural" food could be stuffed with artificial ingredients. "Sugar free" could mean that only one kind of sugar, sucrose, is excluded, but high-calorie sweeteners like honey or corn syrup have been added. Orange juice might be labeled "no preservatives," but orange juice needs no preservatives. Breakfast pastries might be "fortified" with vitamins, but they may also contain a lot of sugar and fat.

The point is you always have to be on the alert at the supermarket. Learn how to read labels and decipher their meanings. Even if it doesn't mean anything to you now, you never know when you might have to do the shopping. And besides, it won't be long until you're on your own.

Health-food stores aren't always "on the up-and-up." Look carefully at food labels for the lowdown on "natural" ingredients.

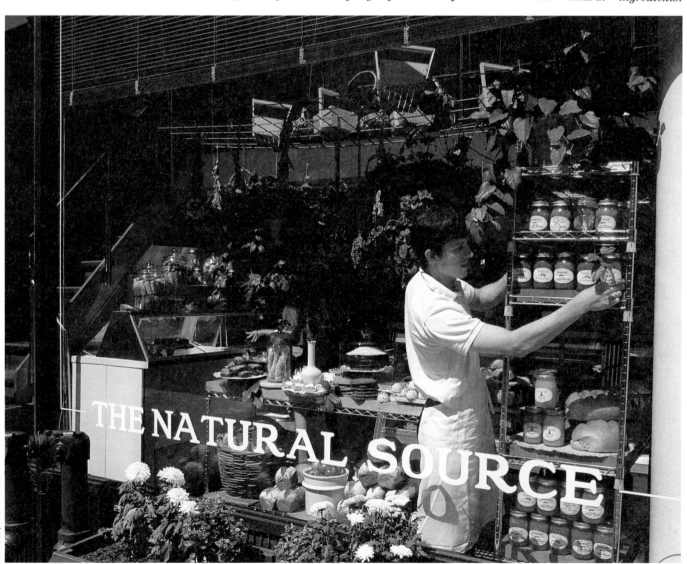

Joe McNally/Wheeler Pictures

THE NATURAL SOURCE

How to Read a Food Label

The Food and Drug Administration requires that *every* food label or package include four pieces of information:

1. The name of the product
2. The net weight
3. The list of ingredients
4. The name of the manufacturer or packer

When a product also makes a nutritional claim (such as "lower in cholesterol") or when the product is enriched or fortified, the label also has to include full nutrition information:

1. Serving size
2. Servings per container
3. Calories per serving
4. Grams of protein, carbohydrates, and fat
5. Cholesterol (if any)
6. Sodium (if any)

And the percentage of the United States Recommended Daily Allowance (USRDA):

1. Amount of protein
2. Amount of different vitamins
3. Amount of different minerals

Perishable foods will include any of the following information:

1. Pack date: the day the food was manufactured or packaged.
2. Pull or sell or freshness date: the last recommended day of sale that allows sufficient time for home storage and use after which the food is not likely to be at its best quality. Example: "Sell by December 27, 1988."
3. Expiration date: the last day the product should be eaten or used for good quality. Example: "Do not use after November 30, 1989."

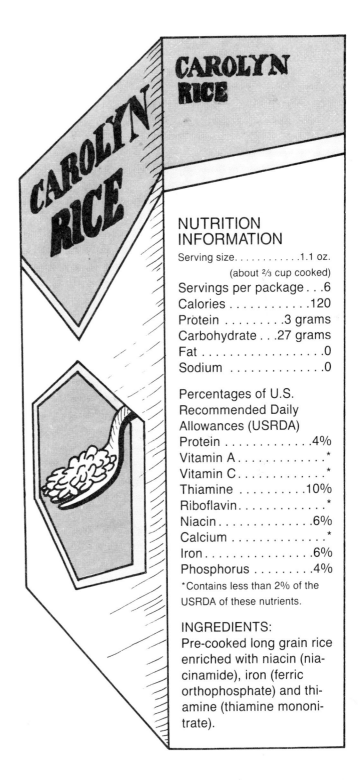

CAROLYN RICE

CAROLYN RICE

NUTRITION INFORMATION

Serving size . . . . 1.1 oz.
(about ⅔ cup cooked)
Servings per package . . . 6
Calories 120
Protein . . . . 3 grams
Carbohydrate . . . 27 grams
Fat 0
Sodium 0

Percentages of U.S. Recommended Daily Allowances (USRDA)
Protein 4%
Vitamin A . . . . *
Vitamin C . . . . *
Thiamine 10%
Riboflavin . . . . *
Niacin 6%
Calcium . . . . *
Iron 6%
Phosphorus 4%
*Contains less than 2% of the USRDA of these nutrients.

INGREDIENTS:
Pre-cooked long grain rice enriched with niacin (niacinamide), iron (ferric orthophosphate) and thiamine (thiamine mononitrate).

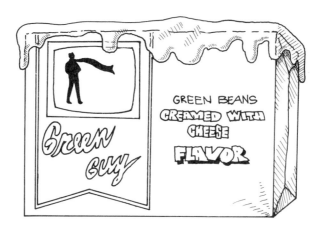

GREEN BEANS
CREAMED WITH CHEESE FLAVOR

Green Guy

Look at a can of food or at the label on page 89.

○ Look at the name and the front of the label. Does it make any claims, like "reduced-calorie" or "no preservatives"? Refer to the list on pages 87–88 to see what that might actually mean.

○ Look at the ingredients. They are listed in order of weight, from the heaviest to the lightest. If sugar is the first ingredient (dextrose, fructose, maltose, and corn syrup are other sugar names), you know it's heavily sweetened. Also look for oils in first or second place. Obviously, the more wholesome foods (spinach, water, enriched whole-wheat flour, and so on) are going to provide the most nutrition.

○ Here's something else to look out for on ingredient lists:

Manufacturers are allowed to use "flexi-labeling." For example: "Contains one or more of the following: sunflower seed oil, coconut oil and/or palm oil." The problem with labeling like this is that the first of these oils is polyunsaturated, while the others contain more saturated fats (definitely the unhealthiest of oils). The polyunsaturated oil is healthier, but you can't be sure it was actually used.

○ Now on to the nutritional information. Although the serving size might seem quite innocent, it, too, can be confusing. These days, manufacturers make servings smaller and smaller to make fat, calories, and sodium levels seem smaller. That sixteen-ounce (480 milliliters) bottle of soda, then, might be divided into two eight-ounce (240 milliliters) servings on the label. The whole can is really 300 calories, not 150.

○ Be sure to take the serving size into consideration when you're comparing different brands. It explains why a four-ounce (120 milliliters) serving of soup has less sodium than an eight-ounce (240 milliliters) serving.

○ Check out the values of protein, carbohydrates, and fat. (The "Fat Formula" on page 92 will help you put some of the information in perspective.)

○ When packaged foods require additional ingredients (skim milk added to cereal; ground beef added to taco sauce), the label may include two nutrition information columns. The first column lists the contents for the package ingredients only. The second lists the nutritional information for the package and the added ingredients together. This makes a big difference when you're figuring out exactly how much you're eating.

○ The U.S. Recommended Daily Allowance (explained in detail on page 60) tells you how good a source this food is for specific nutrients. For example, it says you'll get 6 percent of the protein and 4 percent of the iron you need in one day from two slices of whole-wheat bread.

○ The pack, pull, sell, expiration, or fresh dates should give you an idea of how old the food is and when not to buy or eat it. For example, don't buy milk labeled "September 20" on September 21.

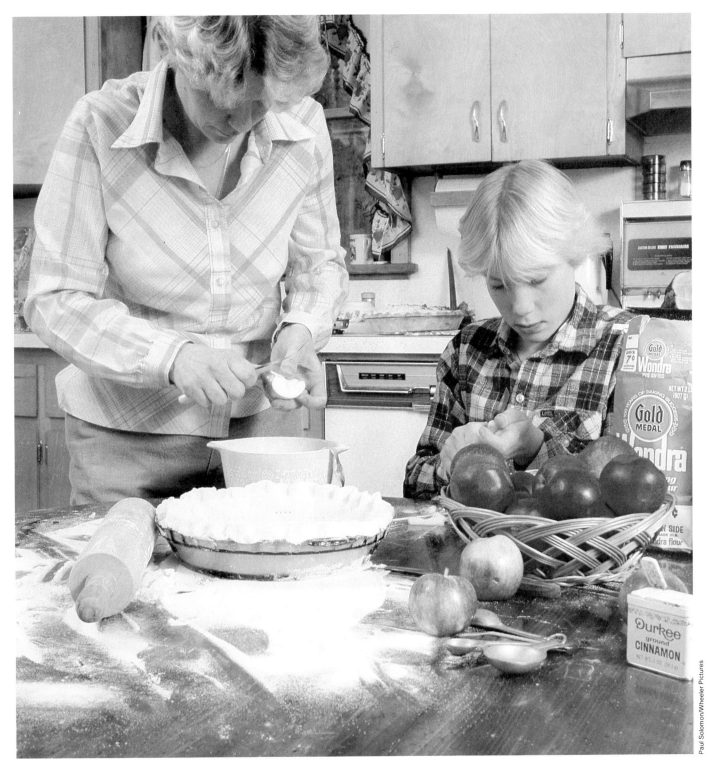

Chances are that an apple pie from a bakery is loaded with fat and sugar. But with help from an adult, you can make desserts with as much as half the undesirable ingredients, while adding whole-wheat flour and chunks of fresh fruits.

at Formula

Food labels tell you the grams of fat in a food serving, but they don't tell you the ratio of fat to other nutrients.

To find the percentage of fat in a processed food, try this formula:

1. Multiply the number of fat grams in one serving by 9 (the number of calories in one gram of fat).
2. Divide the result by the number of calories per serving.
3. Multiply the result by 100.

The answer is the percentage of fat in a serving of food. Here we've tried it with a ½-cup (120-milliliter) serving of chicken noodle soup.

$$2 \text{ grams of fat} \times 9 = 18$$
$$18 \div 70 = 0.205$$
$$.205 \times 100 = 20.5$$

The soup is 20.5% fat.

ealth Foods: *Not Always What They Seem*

Health-food stores are good for finding whole-wheat flours and pasta, dried fruits, tofu, and other foods that are sometimes hard to find in regular supermarkets.

So-called "health foods," however, are not always healthy. As we explained before, the term "natural" can mean most anything on food labels. For instance, granola is often touted as a healthy snack because it's sweetened with "natural" honey. Unfortunately, honey is about as sugary as you can get—even if it is made by bees. Granola is also high in fat and calories.

"Organic" is another term you'll hear. This means that this food has been grown or produced without chemicals. However, leftovers from chemicals used in the environment are found in trace amounts almost anywhere. It's almost impossible to eliminate them altogether.

This isn't to say that health-food stores and healthier foods are completely a hoax. You can find a wealth of good foods (even though they're often more expensive) with these kinds of labels, too. Just be sure that you read the labels and don't simply accept label claims at face value.

Some "Health Foods" (That Aren't)

CAROB CHIPS	BANANA CHIPS
COCONUT MILK	BLACKSTRAP MOLASSES
TOFU FROZEN DESSERTS	NUTS
HONEY	NATURAL POTATO CHIPS
NATURAL PEANUT BUTTER	YOGURT WITH FRUIT PRESERVES

Snacking

You're probably on the run quite a lot, which means that snacking is a daily occurrence . Contrary to what you might have thought before, snacking is a healthy habit. It helps to keep you going and to pack in all the nutrients you need during your busy days. What's more, scientists have found that large meals, as opposed to smaller snacks, might increase your body's levels of insulin, a hormone which may cause your body to store more calories as fat.

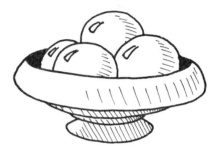

Of course, snacking isn't always beneficial: Snacking on Swiss chocolate rolls, honey-roasted nuts, and fruit candies is going to do more harm than good. Here are good substitutes:

○ Fresh fruits
○ Low-fat vanilla, lemon, or coffee yogurt
○ Whole-wheat fig bars
○ Bran muffins
○ Raisins
○ Frozen grapes and strawberries
○ Unbuttered popcorn
○ Raw vegetables
○ Rye crackers with low-fat cheese
○ Whole-wheat oatmeal cookies
○ Homemade milk shakes (made with skim milk, fruit, and ice)
○ Commercial frozen fruit bars
○ Graham crackers
○ Fruit or vegetable juices
○ Low-fat cottage cheese
○ Low-fat frozen yogurt
○ Low-fat pudding
○ Whole-grain breads

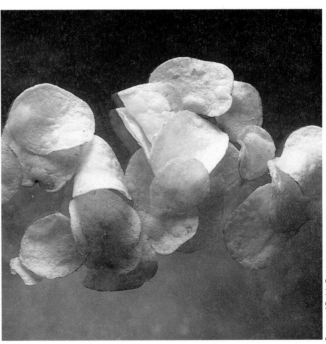

Courtesy of Rodale Press

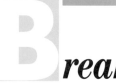 reakfast Boost

You may often skip breakfast because you're running late or you simply don't enjoy breakfast foods, yet research shows time and time again that breakfast is not only nutritionally important, it also helps you perform better. Consider this:

○ In a California study with 7,000 men and women, skipping breakfast was shown to be one among seven different health risks. The health risks all increase the chance of an early death.
○ In a Massachusetts study, breakfast-skipping children were shown to have lesser problem-solving ability.
○ A Minnesota study showed that calories eaten at breakfast helped participants *lose* weight. Calories eaten at night tended to cause weight *gain*.

From reading these surprising facts, it is easy to understand the importance of starting out the day with good nutrition. To be at your best, you simply cannot skip breakfast. After all, your body can't be expected to run well on nothing. (Your last meal was probably about twelve hours before). And remember: The traditional morning meal of eggs and bacon, pancakes and syrup, pre-sweetened cereal, and chocolate milk is not a good choice. Here's a plan for a well-rounded breakfast. Include one food from each category.

Fruit or fruit juice with vitamin C
Orange, tomato, grapefruit, strawberries, cantaloupe.

Protein food
Low-fat milk, cheese, or yogurt; boiled egg or omelet made with one yolk, two whites; turkey or boiled ham.

Cereal or bread
Whole-wheat toast or English muffin; bran muffin; oatmeal or whole-grain cereal.

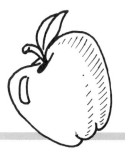
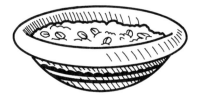
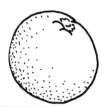

THE FAT FACTS OF CHEESE

Many people mistakenly believe that cheese is a good-for-you food. It's true that cheese is a source of protein, but with a big price to pay in fat intake. The chart below shows this and will help you choose the best kind for the fat price.

CHEESE (1 oz)	CALORIES	FAT (g)	CALCIUM (mg)
American (pasteurized, processed)	106	9	174
cheddar	114	9	204
cream	99	10	23
Edam	101	8	207
Gouda	101	8	198
mozzarella	80	6	147
mozzarella (part-skim)	72	5	183
Muenster	104	9	203
Neufchâtel	74	7	21
provolone	100	8	214
Swiss (natural)	107	8	272
½ cup creamed cottage cheese	117	5	68
½ cup dry-curd cottage cheese	96	.5	36

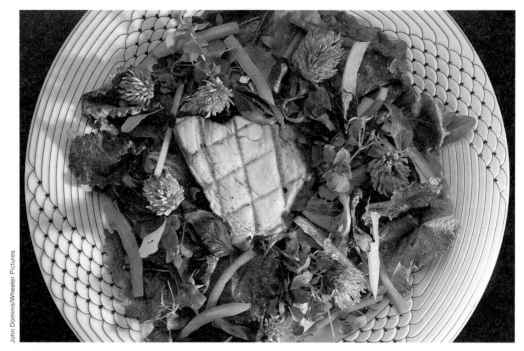

John Dominis/Wheeler Pictures

Order grilled fish in a restaurant, and you can hardly go wrong. Veggies on the side are even better.

Eating Out

The problem with eating out is that you have less control over what goes into your food. Coffee shops and restaurants are one situation; fast-food restaurants are another. At traditional restaurants you can always make special requests, such as having salad dressing served *on the side* of your meal. However, at fast-food restaurants, it is almost impossible to get foods cooked especially to order and with all the fatty, unhealthy aspects of the meal eliminated.

The solutions are to eat at home more often or make the best selections possible.

Restaurants

○ When they're available, choose fresh foods: salads, steamed vegetables, fruit cups, seafood.

○ Don't worry about nibbling on a piece of whole-wheat bread before dinner, but do worry about spreading it with butter.

○ Leave condiments off foods when you can.

○ Don't order menu items described with the following: gravy; fried; au gratin or with cheese sauce; creamed or in cream sauce; buttered or in butter sauce; à la mode; prime.

○ Do order dishes in tomato sauce or with cocktail sauce; stir-fried; poached; garden-fresh; in broth or in its own juice; roasted; steamed.

○ When in doubt, just ask the waiter how something is prepared.

○ Ask if your meat can be broiled or grilled instead of fried.

○ Substitute a baked potato for French fries.

○ Have salad dressings on the side. Vinegar and olive oil or lemon juice are your best choices.

*

It's not easy to choose the most nutritional items when you are eating out. You don't always know what's in a particular dish or how it is prepared. To help you out, we've highlighted the items on this coffee shop menu that are the "safest bets." But don't be afraid to ask what's in something or to tell them how you would like it cooked.

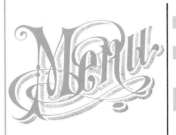

CEREAL
Hot Oatmeal
Cold Cereal (with fresh fruit)

OMELETTES AND EGGS
Two Eggs, Poached or Boiled (served with Toast)
Two Eggs with Bacon, Ham, or Sausage
Plain Omelette
Ham Omelette
Sausage Omelette
Cheese Omelette
Mushroom Omelette

BREADS
Roll, Bagel, Bialy, Toast, English Muffin
Corn, Blueberry, or Bran Muffin

FRUITS AND ASIDES
Half Grapefruit
Half Melon or Wedge of Honeydew
Fresh Fruit Salad
Scoop of Cottage Cheese
Jello (served with Whipped Cream)
Rice Pudding

SOUP
Our Own Soup of the Day
Chili

SALADS
House Salad
Chef's Salad
Spinach Salad
Tuna Salad on a Bed of Lettuce
Individual Can of Tuna on a Bed of Lettuce
Egg Salad on a Bed of Lettuce
Chicken Salad on a Bed of Lettuce
Cottage Cheese and Fruit Salad
Melon and Cottage Cheese

BURGERS
100% Pure Beef Burger, served on a Toasted Bun
Cheeseburger
Pizzaburger

SANDWICHES
Egg Sandwich
Egg and Cheese Sandwich
Egg Salad
Peanut Butter and Jelly
Tuna Salad
Chicken Salad
Bacon, Lettuce, and Tomato
Boiled Ham
Meat Loaf
Roast Beef
Fresh Roast Turkey
Corned Beef

GRILLED SANDWICHES
American Cheese
Swiss Cheese
Cheddar Cheese
Muenster Cheese
Reuben
Tuna Melt

QUICHES
Broccoli and Cheddar Quiche
Spinach, Feta, and Cheddar Quiche

HOT PLATTERS
All Platters served with Hot Vegetable and Baked Potato
Chopped Steak
Hot or Cold Roast Beef or Turkey
Roast Chicken with Stuffing
Virginia Ham Steak
Meatloaf
Eggplant Parmigiana
Lasagna

SIDE ORDERS
Potato Salad or Coleslaw
Baked Potato
Steamed Vegetable of the Day

BEVERAGES
Coffee
Sanka
Tea
Hot Chocolate
Milk
Skim Milk
Chocolate Milk

JUICE BAR
Orange, freshly squeezed
Carrot
V-8
Apple
Pineapple
Grapefruit
Tomato

DESSERTS
Fruit Pies (served a la mode)
Chocolate Layer Cake
Plain Cheese Cake
Fruit Cheese Cake
Donuts
Brownies
Apple Turnover
Carrot Cake
Ice Cream
Ice Cream Shakes
Diet Banana Skim Milk Shake
Diet Fruit Skim Milk Shake

Fast Food

- Watch out for secret sauces—they're usually fatty dressings.
- Order smaller burgers instead of double burgers. Bread is less fatty than meat.
- Instead of cheese, have your burger topped with tomato and lettuce.
- Choose a grilled rather than fried burger.
- Order whole-wheat pizza crusts when you can; have them topped with vegetables.
- When they're available, order broiled fish dinners.
- Baked potatoes are a good choice—but leave off the fatty bacon, cheese, and sour cream toppings. Have it plain, with vegetables, or low-fat yogurt instead.
- Ask for water instead of soda.
- Visit restaurants with salad bars and load up on fresh vegetables. Avoid creamy dressings and mayonnaise-filled salads like potato salad and macaroni salad.
- Choose low-fat frozen yogurt instead of ice cream. Eat it from a cup instead of a sugar cone.
- Remember that the simpler the food, the better it is for you; the extras (sauces, cheeses, extra-crispy batter, butter, syrup, extra burger patties, and so on) usually add fat, sodium, sugar and/or calories.
- Don't fall for the myth that chicken pieces or chicken sandwiches are healthier than burgers; if they're deep-fried, these foods aren't necessarily better.
- Remove the skin from chicken.

A Fast Food Sampler

FOOD	CALORIES	GRAMS OF FAT
McDonald's Big Mac	541	31
Burger King Whopper	606	32
Taco Bell Taco	186	8
Pizza Hut Pepperoni Pizza (½ 10-inch pie)	560	18
Long John Silver's Fish (2 pieces)	318	19
Kentucky Fried Chicken (Original Recipe Dinner)	830	46
Kentucky Fried Chicken (Extra Crispy Dinner)	950	54
Burger King Fries	214	10
McDonald's Egg McMuffin	352	20

Keeping Influence from Friends and Family Under Control

Here's another great way to take charge: Help your friends and family to be as aware of good nutrition as you are. This way they won't be in the way of your good intentions—and they'll be healthier, too.

- Instead of always heading out somewhere to eat, talk your friends into rollerskating, bowling, or seeing a movie.
- Practice your good nutrition habits in front of your friends; you'll be surprised how quickly they catch on.

- Volunteer to go along with whomever does the food shopping in your home. Pass on healthy suggestions.
- Try a little cooking yourself, using all the diet-wise tips you know. You'll not only make a healthier meal, you'll also impress the family—maybe even teach them something new.
- Refill the cookie jars and candy bowls in your home with fresh or dried fruits.
- Don't let your family use food as a reward. Tell them you'd prefer records, clothes, books, magazines—anything but food.
- When you have the chance to pick dinner or dessert, choose something smart.
- Be a good influence on your younger brothers and sisters.

Some parents know about good nutrition—and others don't. Old eating habits—no matter how unhealthy—die hard, so don't expect to make big changes overnight. Food doesn't have to be the center of every family activity. Try exercise instead.

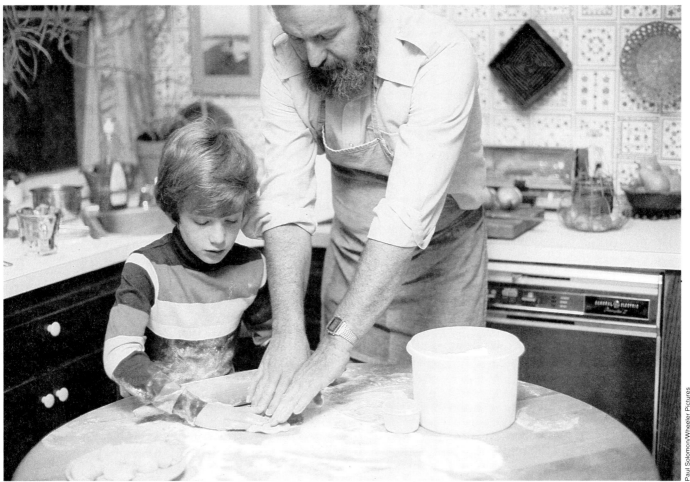

Paul Solomon/Wheeler Pictures

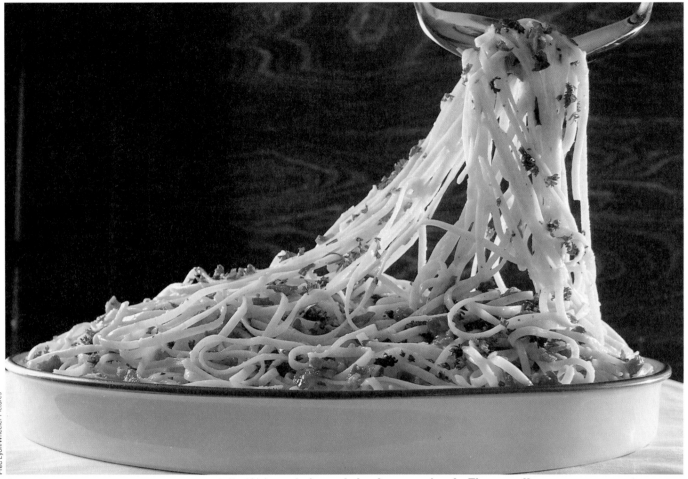

Fred Lyon/Wheeler Pictures

Pasta is a good, nutritional choice especially if it's made from whole wheat or spinach. These noodles are tan or green instead of white, and they taste good, too.

Make a plan for improvement.

This book contains a large chunk of information and advice for you to learn and follow. An easy way to fit it into your life is to set up a week-by-week plan. What follows are suggestions. If you find a way that is better for you, try it!

Every week, add another improvement step. The ones here are general, but they'll accomplish the task when you rely on all the tips you've learned.

Keep a notebook of the foods you eat every day—no matter how small the amount. Before you take on a new step, review it. This helps you realize where you went wrong and where you did well. If you had a particularly hard time fitting in a new habit, then you may decide to work on it for another week before moving on.

When you're ready, move on to the next step.

By the time you reach the end of the plan, you'll be so busy filling your days with nutrient-rich foods, you won't have time for junk foods. And you'll be surprised how much better you feel.

Week 1: Add low-fat proteins.

Week 2: Add low-fat dairy products and cut back on high-fat foods.

Week 3: Add fresh fruits to your daily menu.

Week 4: Add fresh vegetables to your daily menu.

Week 5: Add fresh, steamed, and frozen vegetables without sauces and canned fruit packed in its own juices.

Week 6: Add a daily serving of whole grains.

Week 7: Tie up the loose ends: Drink more water; eliminate excess fats and sugars; eat three meals a day.

Continue to keep your food diary after week 7, aiming for this kind of daily balance:

1. No less than 3 servings of fruit.
   1 serving = 1 medium-sized fresh fruit
   ½ cup (100 grams) canned fruit
   1 glass of fruit juice

2. No less than 3 servings of vegetables.
   1 serving = ½ to 1 cup (100–200 grams) raw or cooked vegetables.

3. No less than 4 servings of whole-grain breads, cereals, pasta, starchy vegetables (corn, potatoes, beans, squash).
   1 serving = 1 slice bread
   ¼–½ cup (50–100 grams) cereal, pasta, vegetables

4. 3 to 4 servings of low-fat milks and cheeses.
   1 serving = 1 8-ounce (240-milliliter) glass of whole milk
   = ½ cup (115 grams) low-fat yogurt or cottage cheese
   = 2 ounces or 2 slices (50 grams) low-fat cheese

5. No more than 7 ounces (200 grams) of lean meat, poultry, seafood.
   7 ounces = 1 small chicken breast and 1 small pork chop
   = 2 slices lean roast beef and ½ cup (115 grams) tuna

Permit yourself an occasional splurge, maybe a ½ cup (120 milliliters) of ice cream or a hot dog once a week. After you follow this plan for a few weeks, it will become a healthy way of life—not an occasional practice. Isn't that the goal you're working toward?

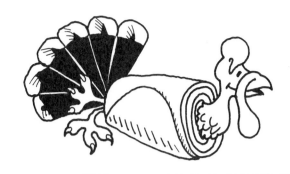

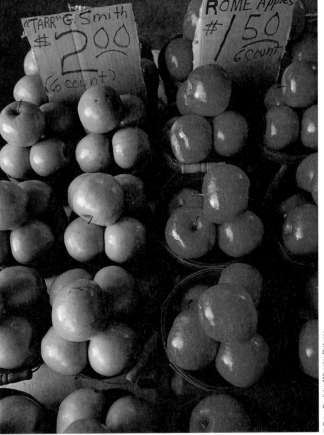

Exercise: *The Role It Plays in Diet*

This book has not fully discussed exercise because it is covered in Volume II, but the bond between nutrition and fitness is strong. Calories, as you know, are the energy food releases into your body. You'll burn some calories by simply reading a book or watching television; it takes calories for all your body functions (heart, digestion, breathing) to function smoothly. You'll burn more calories by walking to school or mopping the floor, because you're using muscles. And you'll burn even more calories by swimming or playing tennis, because you're breathing harder, working your heart harder, and moving your muscles more.

In a nutshell, the reason people get fat is that they eat more calories than their bodies burn. One solution, of course, is to cut back on calories. Another is to increase exercise. The best answer of all: Cut calories and increase your exercise regimen.

Even if you aren't on a weight-loss plan, exercise helps your body burn calories efficiently. It's a relationship we can't ignore. (For more on the healthy benefits of exercise, see ''Exercise.'') This chart will give you some idea of how calories are used.

ACTIVITY	CALORIES BURNED PER MINUTE
Sleeping	1
Studying	2.2
Piano playing	3.2
Walking	5.4
Bicycling	6.7
Lawnmowing	7.7
Rollerskating (fast)	11.2
Ropeskipping	13.3
Cross-country skiing	16.7

TO BURN OFF:	IT TAKES:
1 12-ounce (350 milliliter) soda	39 minutes of badminton
1 hot fudge sundae	66 minutes of fast-paced aerobic dancing
1 piece homemade chocolate meringue pie	96 minutes of woodchopping
1 ham-and-cheese omelet	103 minutes of tennis
3 piece order of fried fish	153 minutes of stationary bike riding
1 fast food double burger with cheese	238 minutes half-court basketball

How can you tell if a sport rates high in the exercise department? Use your head. If leg and arm power are utilized, you're getting a good workout. Sorry, but motorized dirt bikes don't count.

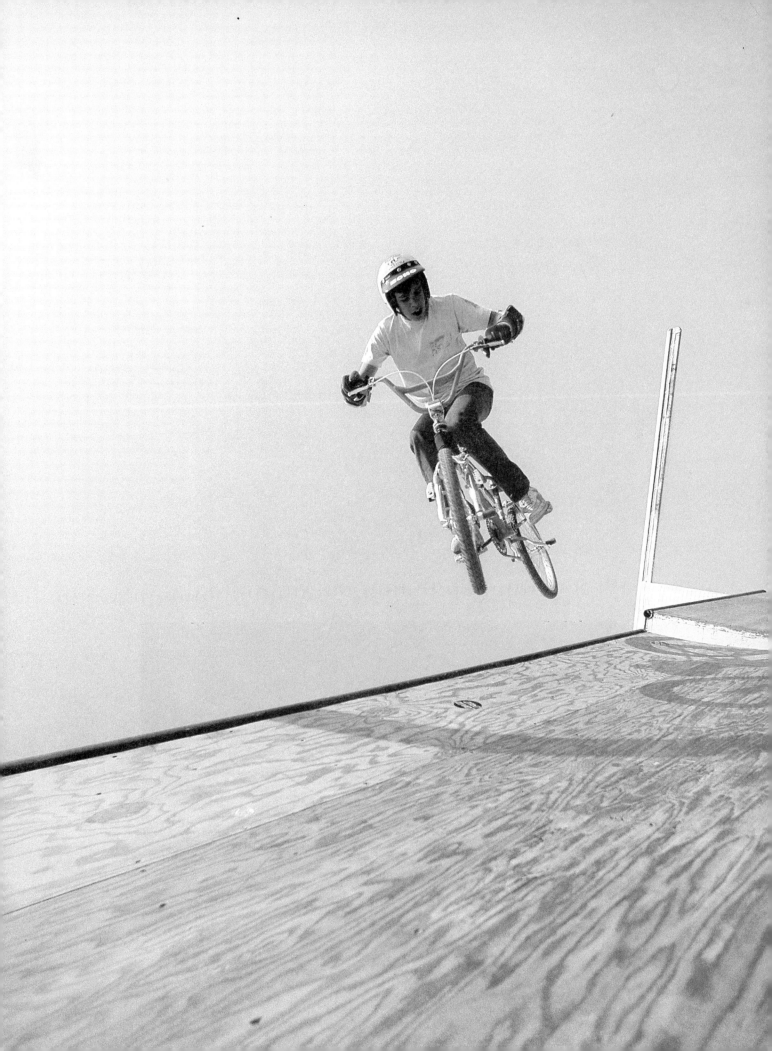

Fat Content

This chart tells you how many tablespoons of fat in each of these foods.

1 3½" bagel 1 c. cocoa with skim milk	= ½ ×
1 slice cheese pizza (5½" arc)	= 1 ×
2 2½" chocolate-chip cookies 10 potato chips	= 2 ×
10 french fries 1 oz. peanuts or cashews	= 3 ×
3 oz. cheeseburger with 1 slice American cheese 1½-oz. hot dog with roll	= 4 ×
6 chicken nuggets 1 c. macaroni and cheese	= 5 ×
Bacon cheeseburger with 1 slice cheese, 2 slices bacon 1 slice pecan pie (⅛ of an 8" pie)	= 6 ×
1 grilled cheese sandwich with 2 slices cheese 1 slice strawberry shortcake (⅛ of an 8" cake)	= 7 ×
Fast-food fried fish sandwich Sandwich with slices of ham, cheese, 2 t. mayo	= 8 ×

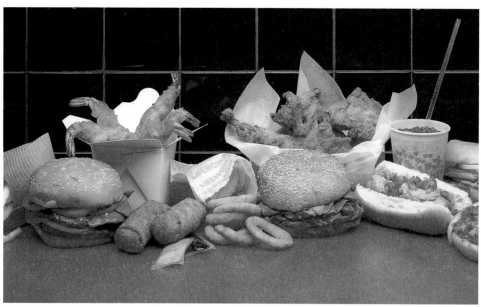

Courtesy of Rodale Press

You're On Your Own!

Quick! What's the difference between a simple carbohydrate and a complex carbohydrate? Anorexia nervosa and bulimia? A "quack" diet and a nutritional diet?

Don't feel bad if the answers aren't on the tip of your tongue. It's not important that you're able to cite facts and figures at a moment's notice. But it is important for you to fit good nutrition into your daily patterns. You can do that by making the right food choices, carefully watching over your health, and steering clear of bad influences.

Can you do it? Of course, but it takes know-how—and sometimes discipline. It is, however, a challenge worth taking. But remember: If you get confused or forget how to handle a nutritional dilemma, this book is always here to help.

Nutritional charts

FOOD ITEM	MEASURE	CALORIES	CARBO–HYDRATES g	PROTEIN g	TOTAL FAT g	CHOLESTEROL mg	SODIUM mg	CALCIUM mg
BEVERAGES								
Coffee, clear	1 cup	5	.8	.3	.1		2.3	4.6
Cola drinks	1 cup	94	19	0	0		2	
Fruit-flavored drinks	1 cup	110	29	0	0		18	
Diet drinks	1 cup	t		0	0		50	
Tea, clear	1 cup	4	.9	.1	t		1.6	5
BREADS, FLOURS, CEREALS, GRAINS, AND GRAIN PRODUCTS								
Bran flakes, 40%, fortified	1 cup	106	28.2	3.6	.6		207	19
Breads								
Biscuit, enr	2″ diam.	103	12.8	2.1	4.8		175	34
Cornbread	2″ sq	93	13.1	3.3	3.2	30	283	54
Pumpernickel	1 slice	79	17	2.9	.4		182	27
White, enr	1 slice	62	11.6	2	.79		117	20
Whole wheat	1 slice	56	11	2.4	.7		121	23
Cornflakes, fortified	1 cup	97	21	2	.1		251	1–7
Crackers								
Graham, plain	1 lg	55	10.4	1.1	1.3		95	6
Whole wheat, Ak-Mak	4 pieces	117	18.9	4.64	2.33			21.3
Muffins								
Bran, enr	1 avg	104	17.2	3.1	3.9		179	57
Corn meal, whl grd	1 med	130	19.1	3.2	4.6		223	50
Oatmeal (rolled oats), ckd	1 cup	132	23.3	4.8	2.4		.8	22
Pancakes								
Plain, enr	4″ diam	62	9.2	1.9	1.9		115	27
Whole wheat	4″ diam	74	8.8	3.4	3.2			50
Pasta, whole wheat, dry	4 oz.	400	78	20	1			20
Pizza, cheese, 14″ diam	⅛	153	18.4	7.8	5.4		456	144

Nutritional charts

FOOD ITEM	MEASURE	CALORIES	CARBO—HYDRATES g	PROTEIN g	TOTAL FAT g	CHOLESTEROL mg	SODIUM mg	CALCIUM mg
Popcorn, plain	1 cup	54	10.7	1.8	.7		t	2
Rice								
Brown, ckd w/salt	1 cup	178	38.2	3.8	1.2		423	18
White, ckd w/salt	1 cup	223	49.6	4.1	.4		767	21
Spaghetti, enr, ckd	1 cup	155	32.2	4.8	.6		1	11
Waffles, plain, enr	5½″ diam	209	28.1	7	7.4		356	85
Wheat flakes, fortified	1 cup	106	24.2	3.1	.72		310	12
DAIRY PRODUCTS								
Cheese								
American, pasteurized, processed	1 oz	107	.5	6.5	8.86	27	406	174
Cheddar, American	1 oz	112	.36	7	9.4	30	176	211
Cheese spread, American, pasteurized, processed	1 oz	81	2.3	4.5	6	16	381	158
Cottage, creamed, not packed	1 cup	217	5.6	26.2	9.47	31	850	126
Cottage, 2% fat, not packed	1 cup	203	8.2	31	4.36	19	918	155
Mozzarella	1 oz	80	.63	5.51	6.12	22	106	147
Mozzarella, part skim, low moisture	1 oz	79	.89	7.79	4.85	15	150	207
Ricotta, whl milk	1 cup	428	7.48	27.7	31.9	124	207	509
Ricotta, part skim	1 cup	340	12.6	28	19.5	9	307	669
Swiss	1 oz	107	.96	8.06	7.78	26	74	272
Egg								
Fried	1 lg	99	.53	5.37	6.4	312	144	26
Hard cooked	1 lg	82	.5	6.5	5.8	312	61	27
Poached	1 lg	82	.5	6.5	5.8	312	61	27
Ice cream, hard	1 cup	269	31.7	4.8	14.3	59	116	176
Ice milk, hard	1 cup	184	29	5.16	5.63	18	105	176

Nutritional charts

FOOD ITEM	MEASURE	CALORIES	CARBO—HYDRATES g	PROTEIN g	TOTAL FAT g	CHOLESTEROL mg	SODIUM mg	CALCIUM mg
Milk								
Chocolate, whole	1 cup	208	25.9	7.92	8.48	30	149	280
Low-fat	1 cup	121	11.7	8.12	4.68	18	122	297
Skim	1 cup	86	11.8	8.35	.44	4	126	302
Whole	1 cup	159	11.4	8.5	8.15	33	120	291
Yogurt								
Whole milk, plain	8 oz	139	10.6	7.88	7.38	29	105	274
Low-fat, plain, 12 g protein	8 oz	144	16	11.9	3.52	14	159	415
DESSERTS AND SWEETS								
Brownies, enr, 2 × 2 × ¾″	1 piece	146	15.3	2	9.4	25.5	75	12
Cake								
Chocolate, devils food, no icing, 2 × 3 × 2″	1 piece	165	23.4	2.2	7.7		132	33
Pound, old-fashioned, 3 × 3 × ½″	1 piece	142	14.1	1.7	8.8		33	6
Cake Icing								
Chocolate	1 cup	1034	185	8.8	38.2		168	165
White, boiled	1 cup	297	75.5	1.3	0		134	2
Candy								
Caramel, plain or chocolate	1 piece	20	3.88	.2	.536		11.4	7.5
Chocolate milk bar, plain	1 oz	147	16.1	2.2	9.2		27	65
Chocolate syrup	1 tbsp	46	11.7	.45	.49		10	3
Cookies								
Chocolate chip, enr, 2⅓″ diam	1	51	6	.55	3		34.8	3.5
Oatmeal w/raisin, 3″ diam	1	63	10.3	.9	2.2		23	3
Doughnut								
Cake, plain	1 avg	125	16.4	1.5	6		160	13
Jellies	1 tbsp	49	12.7	t	t		3	4

Nutritional charts

FOOD ITEM	MEASURE	CALORIES	CARBO—HYDRATES g	PROTEIN g	TOTAL FAT g	CHOLESTEROL mg	SODIUM mg	CALCIUM mg
Pie								
Apple, 1/6 of 9" pie	1 piece	410	61	3.4	17.8	156	482	1
Pecan, 1/6 of pie	1 piece	668	82	8.2	36.6		354	75
Pumpkin, 1/6 of pie	1 piece	317	36.7	6	16.8	91	321	76
Pudding								
Bread w/raisins, enr	1 cup	496	75.3	14.8	16.2	170	533	289
Chocolate, cornstarch	1 cup	385	66.8	8.1	12.2	30	146	250
FISH AND SEAFOOD								
Catfish	1 lb	467	0	79.8	14.1		272	
Flounder, sole, or sandabs	1 lb	358	0	75.8	5.44	227	354	54
Salmon								
Fresh	1 lb	984	0	102	60.8	272	217	358
Pink, canned	1 cup	310	0	45.1	13	77	851	431
Shrimp, fresh	1 lb	413	6.8	82.1	3.6	680	635	286
Trout, rainbow	1 lb	885	0	97.5	51.7	249	177	86
Tuna								
Canned in oil, drained	1 cup	315	0	46.1	13.1	104		13
Canned in water	1 cup	254	0	56	1.6	126	82	32
Whitefish	1 lb	703	0	85.7	37.2		236	
FRUITS AND JUICES								
Apple								
Raw	1 med	96	24	.3	1		2	12
Juice, unsw	1 cup	117	29.5	.2	t		2	15
Banana, raw	1 avg	127	33.3	1.6	.3		2	12
Blackberries, raw	1 cup	84	18.6	1.7	1.3		1	46
Cantaloupe, raw	1/4 avg	30	7.5	.7	.1		12	14
Cherries								

Nutritional charts

FOOD ITEM	MEASURE	CALORIES	CARBO—HYDRATES g	PROTEIN g	TOTAL FAT g	CHOLESTEROL mg	SODIUM mg	CALCIUM mg
Sour, raw, pitted	1 cup	90	22.2	1.9	.5		3	34
Sour, canned, hvy syrup	1 cup	119	29.6	2.2	.5		2	37
Grapes								
American (slip skin) raw	1 cup	106	24	2	1.5		5	24
Honeydew melon, raw	2″ wide	49	11.5	1.2	.5		18	21
Lemonade, frozen concentrate, diluted	1 cup	107	28.3	.1	t		1	2
Olives								
Green	2 med	15	.2	.2	1.6		312	8
Ripe	2 lg	37	.6	.2	4		150	21
Greek (salt-cured)	3 med	67	1.7	.4	7.1		658	
Peach								
Raw	1 med	38	9.7	.6	.1		1	9
Canned, hvy syrup	1 cup	200	51.5	1	.3		5	10
Pear								
Raw	1 avg	122	30.6	1.4	.8		4	16
Canned, hvy syrup	1 cup	194	50	.5	.5		3	13
Pineapple								
Diced, raw	1 cup	81	21.2	.6	.3		2	26
Canned, hvy syrup	1 cup	189	49.5	.8	.3		3	28
Raisins, packed	1 cup	477	128	4.1	.3		45	102
Strawberries								
Raw	1 cup	56	12.6	1	.8		2	32
Frozen, sweetened, unthawed	1 cup	278	70.9	1.3	.5		3	36
Watermelon, slice	6″ × 1½″	156	38.4	3	1.2		6	42
MEAT AND POULTRY								
Beef								

Nutritional charts

FOOD ITEM	MEASURE	CALORIES	CARBO—HYDRATES g	PROTEIN g	TOTAL FAT g	CHOLESTEROL mg	SODIUM mg	CALCIUM mg
Chuck roast	1 lb	905	0	78.8	75	270	276	49
Flank steak	1 lb	653	0	98	25.9	261	343	59
Ground beef, lean	1 lb	812	0	93.9	45.4	295		54
Ground beef, regular	1 lb	1216	0	81.2	96.2	307		45
Liver	1 lb	635	24	90.3	17.3	1360	617	36
Sirloin steak	1 lb	1316	0	71	112	261	249	42
Chicken								
Breast	1 lb	394	0	74.5	18	239	377	39
Drumstick	1 lb	313	0	51.2	30.7	239	377	35
Thigh	1 lb	435	0	61.6	33.5	368	377	41
Wing	1 lb	325	0	41.1	52.7	368	377	22
Chili con carne w/beans	1 cup	339	31	19	15.6		1354	82
Frankfurter	1 lb	1402	8.2	56.7	131	295	4990	32
Lamb, leg	1 lb	845	0	67.7	61.7	265	237	39
Pork								
Bacon, sliced	1 lb	3016	4.5	38.1	314	999	3084	59
Chops	1 lb	1065	0	61	89	260	214	36
Ham, cured	1 lb	1535	1.2	66.7	138	318	3415	41
Potted meat, all kinds	1 lb	558	0	39.4	43.2		137	22
Bologna	1 lb	1379	5	54.9	133		5897	32
Salami	1 lb	2041	5.4	108	151			64
Turkey								
Dark meat, ckd	1 lb	921	0	136	37.6	458	449	36
Light meat, ckd	1 lb	798	0	149	17.7	349	372	36
Veal (calf), Cutlet	1 lb	681	0	72.3	41	254	253	41
NUTS, NUT PRODUCTS, AND SEEDS								
Almonds, raw	1 cup	849	27.7	26.4	77		6	332

Nutritional charts

FOOD ITEM	MEASURE	CALORIES	CARBO—HYDRATES g	PROTEIN g	TOTAL FAT g	CHOLESTEROL mg	SODIUM mg	CALCIUM mg
Cashews, roasted	1 cup	785	41	24.1	64		21	53
Peanuts, roasted	1 cup	838	29.7	37.7	70.1		7	104
Pecans, halves, raw	1 cup	742	15.8	9.9	76.9		t	79
OILS, FATS, AND SHORTENING								
Butter	1 tbsp	102	.1	.1	11.5	35	2240	45
Margarine								
Regular	1 tbsp	102	.1	.1	11.5	0	140	3
Whipped	1 tbsp	68	t	.1	7.6	0	93	2
Oils								
Corn	1 tbsp	126	0	0	14	t	t	t
Olive	1 tbsp	124	t	t	14	t	.001	.07
Peanut	1 tbsp	124	t	t	14	t	t	t
Safflower	1 tbsp	124	0	0	14	t	t	t
Sunflower	1 tbsp	124	t	t	14	t	t	t
SALAD DRESSINGS AND SAUCES								
Barbecue sauce	1 tbsp	14	1.25	.238	1.08		127	3.3
Catsup, tomato	1 tbsp	16	3.8	3	.1		156	3
Mayonnaise	1 tbsp	101	.3	.2	11.2	10	84	3
Mustard	1 tbsp	15	.9	.9	.9		195	18
Salad dressings								
French, regular	1 tbsp	66	2.8	.1	6.2		219	2
French, low calorie	1 tbsp	15	2.5	.1	.7		126	2
Italian	1 tbsp	83	1	t	9		314	2
Thousand Island, regular	1 tbsp	80	2.5	.1	8		112	2
Thousand Island, low calorie	1 tbsp	27	2.3	.1	2.1		105	2
Soy sauce	1 tbsp	12	1.7	1	.2		1319	15
Vinegar	1 tbsp	2	.9	t	0		t	1

Nutritional charts

FOOD ITEM	MEASURE	CALORIES	CARBO — HYDRATES g	PROTEIN g	TOTAL FAT g	CHOLESTEROL mg	SODIUM mg	CALCIUM mg
SOUPS								
Chicken noodle	1 cup	62	7.9	3.4	1.9		979	10
Clam chowder								
Manhattan	1 cup	81	12.3	2.2	2.5		938	34
New England	1 cup	130	10.5	4.3	7.7		104	91
Mushroom, cream of	1 cup	134	10.1	2.4	9.6		955	41
Pea, split	1 cup	145	20.6	8.6	3.2		941	29
Turkey noodle	1 cup	79	8.4	4.3	2.9		998	14
Vegetable								
Beef	1 cup	78	9.6	5.1	2.2		1046	12
Vegetarian	1 cup	78	13.2	2.2	2		838	20
VEGETABLES, LEGUMES, SPROUTS, AND VEGETABLE JUICES								
Beans								
Black-eye peas, ckd	1 cup	178	29.9	13.4	1.3		2	40
Canned w/pork	1 cup	304	47.6	15.2	6.4		1158	136
Green, snap, ckd	1 cup	31	6.8	2	.3		5	63
Green, snap, canned, drained	1 cup	32	7	1.9	.3		319	61
Lima, ckd	1 cup	262	48.6	15.6	1.1		4	55
Lima, canned, drained	1 cup	163	31	9.2	.5		401	48
Pinto, dry	1 cup	663	121	43.5	2.3		19	257
Red kidney, ckd	1 cup	218	39.6	14.4	.9		6	70
Red kidney, canned	1 cup	230	41.8	14.5	1		8	74
Broccoli								
Raw, 5½″ long	1 piece	32	5.9	3.6	.3		15	103
Cooked	1 cup	40	7	4.8	.5		16	136
Brussels sprouts, cooked	1 cup	56	9.9	6.5	.6		16	50
Cabbage, common, sliced, ckd	1 cup	29	6.2	1.6	.3		20	64

Nutritional charts

FOOD ITEM	MEASURE	CALORIES	CARBO— HYDRATES g	PROTEIN g	TOTAL FAT g	CHOLESTEROL mg	SODIUM mg	CALCIUM mg
Carrots								
Raw	1 lg	42	9.7	1.1	.2			
Cooked	1 cup	48	11	1.4	.3		47	37
Canned, drained	1 cup	47	10.4	1.2	.5		51	51
Celery, raw	1 cup	20	4.7	1.1	.1		151	47
Corn								
Cooked	1 cup	137	31	5.3	1.7		t	5
Canned, drained	1 cup	139	32.7	4.3	1.3		389	8
Cream-style canned	1 cup	210	51.2	5.4	1.5		604	8
Lettuce								
Boston or bibb, raw	1 cup	8	1.4	.7	.1		5	19
Iceberg, raw	1 cup	10	2.2	.7	.1		7	15
Mushrooms								
Raw	1 cup	20	3.1	1.9	.2		11	4
Onions								
Raw	1 cup	65	14.8	2.6	.2		17	46
Cooked	1 cup	61	13.7	2.5	.2		15	50
Peas								
Cooked	1 cup	114	19.4	8.6	.6		2	37
Canned, drained	1 cup	150	28.6	8	.7		401	44
Split, ckd	1 cup	230	41.6	16	.3		26	22
Peppers, green, sliced, raw	1 cup	18	3.8	1	.2		10	7
Pickles								
Dill	1 lg	11	2.2	.7	.4		1428	26
Sweet (gherkins)	1 lg	51	12.8	.2	.1			4
Potatoes								
Baked in skin	1 lg	145	32.8	4	.2		6	14

Nutritional charts

FOOD ITEM	MEASURE	CALORIES	CARBO— HYDRATES g	PROTEIN g	TOTAL FAT g	CHOLESTEROL mg	SODIUM mg	CALCIUM mg
French fries	10 pieces	137	18	2.1	6.6		379	26
Hash browns	1 cup	355	45.1	4.8	18.1			
Mashed w/milk	1 cup	137	27.3	4.4	1.5		446	19
Scalloped and au gratin w/cheese	1 cup	355	33.3	13	19.4	36	1095	311
Potato chips	10 chips	113	10	1.1	8		95	8
Spinach								
Cooked	1 cup	41	6.5	5.4	.5		90	167
Canned, drained	1 cup	49	7.4	5.5	1.2		484	242
Sweet potato								
Baked	1 avg	161	37	2.4	.6		14	46
Candied, 2″ × 4″	2 halves	168	34.2	1.3	3.3		42	37

GLOSSARY

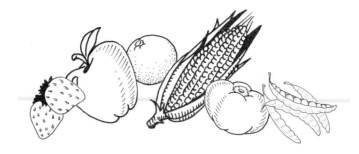

Additives Chemical or food substances added to food products for different purposes: (1) to fortify, or make foods healthier; (2) to preserve, or keep foods from spoiling; (3) to add flavor.

Allspice A sweet, highly scented, hot spice often added to sausages, pickles, fish dishes, and tomato-juice cocktails.

Anorexia nervosa An eating disorder characterized by a person's refusal to eat normal amounts of food in order to lose weight. The result: The victim becomes unhealthily thin and, perhaps, malnourished.

Appetite The desire to eat and feed your body.

Artery A large vessel carrying blood from the heart to various parts of the body.

Artificial sweeteners Sweet-tasting chemicals that replace the sugar in food. Generally, artificial sweeteners add sweetness to food without adding as many calories.

Bake To cook food in dry heat, usually in an oven.

Blood The fluid that circulates in the heart and vessels of vertebrate animals, carrying food and oxygen to, and waste from, all parts of the body.

Boil To cook food in a liquid (usually water) in which the bubbles break on the surface and steam rises.

Broil To cook food by exposing it to direct heat under a very hot flame or over hot coals.

Broth A clear soup.

Bulimia An eating disorder in which a person frequently forces himself to vomit in order to lose weight. Eventually, he gets sick because he isn't taking in enough nutrients.

Caffeine A stimulating substance found in foods (chocolate, candy), beverages (cocoa, coffee, tea, soda), and medicines (pain relievers, allergy remedies, alertness tablets). It occurs naturally in the leaves, seeds, or fruits of various plants, such as cocoa beans and kola nuts. When you eat or drink a caffeinated food, you feel more alert or "jittery," because caffeine works on your central nervous system, heart, muscles, and stomach.

Calcium A mineral that supports the growth and strength of bones and teeth, holds cells together, and helps the blood clot. Some good sources of calcium are: low-fat dairy foods, green, leafy vegetables, sardines, and other canned fish.

Calorie A measurement of how much energy a food produces. When we eat too many calories, the body stores the excess in fat cells. Only carbohydrates, protein, and fat make calories.

GLOSSARY

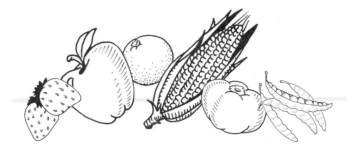

Cancer A collection of dangerous diseases that are alike in that they all grow fast and are hard to control. One of the most common forms is cancer of the colon (part of the large intestine through which waste passes), which may be caused by fatty foods.

Carbohydrates A nutrient that provides energy for the body. Some carbohydrates are complex, such as fruits, vegetables, and whole-grain foods. Others are simple, such as sugar and sugary foods.

Cardamom A sweet, strong, lemon-flavored spice. Cardamom is often used in baked goods.

Cell The microscopic, basic building block that makes up the entire human body.

"Choice" meat A United States Department of Agriculture label identifying meat with a fat percentage higher than "good," "lean," and "extra lean" meat.

Cholesterol A waxy, fat-like substance found only in foods from animals, such as dairy foods, eggs, and meat. Cholesterol is also made by the liver to help manufacture cell membranes, hormones, vitamin D, and other essential nutrients. Even though cholesterol is necessary for healthiness, after six months of age it is not necessary to have external sources of cholesterol.

Chromium A mineral that helps the body break down and use carbohydrates.

Cinnamon A warm, fragrant spice found mostly in two forms: Sticks are used in pickling as well as to spice coffee and pudding. Cinnamon is sprinkled on puddings, hot cereals, apple pie, and other baked foods.

Clove A strong spice often used to flavor ham, pork, pies, puddings, and other baked goods.

Complex carbohydrates A nutrient that provides energy. It is found in plant foods such as potatoes, beans, corn, wheat bread, pasta, and bran cereal. Complex carbohydrates are also known as "starch."

Condiments Any substance added to food at the table, such as salt, vinegar, ketchup, soy sauce, and Worcestershire sauce.

Constipation The abnormally slow passage, or halt, of bowel movements.

Copper A mineral that helps blood do its job. Some good sources of copper are: nuts, cocoa powder, raisins, and dried beans.

Croissant A crescent-shaped roll.

Deep fry To cook food by "soaking" in hot fat or oil.

GLOSSARY

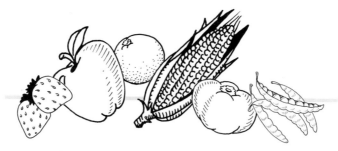

Diabetes (diabetes mellitus) A collection of diseases resulting from the lack of insulin, a chemical involved in feeding the cells. A person doesn't "catch" diabetes, but is born with a tendency to develop this disease. One type is found mostly in overweight adults, another in people under the age of 25. If a diabetic watches his diet very carefully, he may have few problems with this disease.

Diarrhea The abnormal passage of frequent and loose, watery, bowel movements.

Dietary Guidelines for Americans A plan of healthy eating habits established by the United States Department of Agriculture and the United States Department of Health and Human Services.

Disease Harmful disorders in the body. You can "catch" a disease from someone or something, be born with one, or help cause it with certain health habits. For example, eating or not eating certain foods can increase the risk of getting cancer.

Ectomorph One of the three basic body types.

Endomorph One of the three basic body types.

"Enriched" products The addition of certain nutrients lost in foods during processing and refining.

Esophagus The tube through which food passes from the mouth to the stomach.

"Extra lean" meat A United States Department of Agriculture label identifying meat with the least percentage of fat, compared to "prime," "choice," "good," and "lean."

Fat (1) Dietary fat is the fat found in food; it could be hidden inside a hot dog, or be as obvious as butter or oil. Dietary fat is very high in calories, takes longer to digest than other nutrients, and is one of the nutrients we need very little of. People who eat a lot of fat are likely to have health problems such as obesity, cancer, and heart disease. (2) Body fat is the layer of cells beneath the skin. Some body fat is necessary for keeping us warm and cushioning our organs. Some people, however, eat too much dietary fat or high-calorie, sugary foods, and since the body stores extra calories when it exceeds the number it needs for energy, there is a body fat excess.

Fiber A food substance found in complex carbohydrates. It is the undigestable cell walls of plants. Fiber is good because it "bulks up" body waste and helps it leave our system faster. In the process, it takes and scrapes away any fatty, cancer-causing substances. Examples of fibrous foods are apples, whole-wheat products, broccoli, and beans.

GLOSSARY

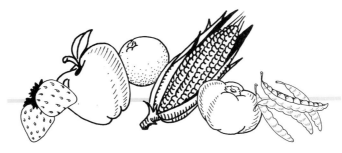

Fibrocystic breast disease A non-cancerous, "lumpy breast" condition found in women, particularly as they get older.

Flexi-labeling A label identifying more than one ingredient that may have been added to a product. Example: "Contains one or more of the following: sunflower seed oil, coconut oil and/or palm oil."

Fluoride A mineral that helps prevent tooth decay. Fluoride may also help prevent the loss of bone structure with age. Some good sources of fluoride are fish, most low-fat animal foods, and tea.

Food & Drug Administration (FDA) A United States government agency that tests and approves or rejects food products for the market.

"Fortified" products Foods with nutrients added beyond natural levels.

Fry To cook food rapidly in an open pan with a large amount of fat or oil.

"Good" meat A United States Department of Agriculture label identifying meat with a fat percentage higher than "lean" and "extra lean" meat, but lower than "prime" or "choice."

Ginger A peppery spice that can be found in relishes, Japanese food, ginger snaps, gingerbread, and other baked goods.

Grill To cook food over hot coals or under a broiler.

Hard cheeses Cheddar, Parmesan, Romano, Gruyere, Swiss, sapsago, spalen, curd.

Heartburn A burning discomfort in the chest; usually a result of digestive problems.

Heart disease A disorder affecting the heart. A person may be born with heart disease or he may have certain health habits that increase the risk of this problem (see "Exercise").

Hormone Natural chemicals in the body that control various functions, from growth to urination (see "Sex and Hormonal Changes").

Indigestion Difficulty in digesting certain foods, which results in an uncomfortable sensation, heartburn, gas, or belching.

Intestines (small and large) Organs that help break down food so it can be absorbed into the bloodstream. They are located behind the stomach wall.

Iodine A mineral that helps the thyroid gland function. Some good sources of iodine are seafood, and table salt.

GLOSSARY

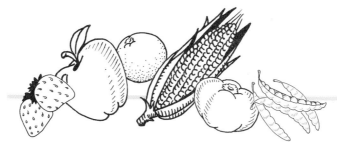

Iron A mineral that helps blood carry oxygen through the body and release energy from food. Some good sources of iron are: whole-grain foods, eggs, dried beans, and low-fat meats.

Kiwi A New Zealand fruit about the size of a large plum, fuzzy brown on the outside and bright green inside. Its flavor is sweetly sour.

Large intestine See Intestines

Laxative A food or drug that forces frequent bowel movements.

"Leaner" meat A label identifying meat as a product with twenty-five percent less fat or cholesterol as compared to United States Department of Agriculture's standards for that product.

"Lean" meat (1) A United States Department of Agriculture label identifying meat with a fat percentage higher than "extra lean," but lower than "prime," "choice," or "good." (2) A label identifying meat with 10 percent less fat and cholesterol as compared to United States Department of Agriculture standards for that product.

Legumes Dried beans and peas, such as pinto beans, black-eyed peas, soybeans, navy beans, and snap peas.

"Lite" or "light" (1) A label identifying meat as a product with twenty-five percent less fat or cholesterol as compared to United States Department of Agriculture standards for that product. (2) Foods that may have fewer calories than their comparable products. *Not* controlled by the United States Department of Agriculture or the Food & Drug Administration.

"Low-calorie" A Food & Drug Administration (FDA) label identifying a product that has no more than forty calories per serving.

"Low fat" (1) A label identifying meat with ten percent less fat and cholesterol as compared to United States Department of Agriculture standards for that product. (2) Any product with a reduction in the normal percentage of fat.

Low-fat milk Milk with some fat removed, compared to whole milk, which has the most fat, and skim milk, which has the least amount of fat possible.

"Lower fat" meat A label identifying meat as a product with twenty-five percent less fat or cholesterol as compared to United States Department of Agriculture standards for that product.

Magnesium A mineral that helps nerves and muscles function properly. Some good sources of magnesium are low-fat meat, fish, and whole-grain foods.

GLOSSARY

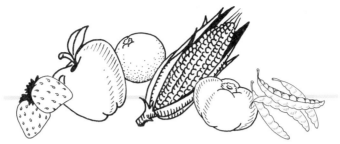

Malnutrition A condition in which a person becomes sick because he isn't getting enough nutrients. Not only is a malnourished person more susceptible to other diseases, but he may also be extremely underweight and have pale, scaly, swollen, or red skin; bleeding gums; and dull, brittle hair.

Mannitol A natural sweetener found in pineapple, olives, carrots, asparagus, and other foods. It is used in many manufactured foods as a preservative or additive.

Maraschino cherries Bright-red cherries packaged in a strong, sweet liquid.

Menstruation The first part of a female's monthly reproductive cycle, when blood passes through the vagina (in the genital area) if the female is not pregnant.

Mesomorph One of the three basic body types.

Mineral water Bottled water that contains dissolved minerals.

Minerals An element found in food or made by the body, necessary for normal growth and function.

Monosaturated fat Fat that has very little effect on cholesterol, but like all other fats, is high in calories. Monosaturated fat is found in peanut, olive, and rice oils.

Muscles A body tissue that contracts and produces motion.

Niacin Vitamins B1 and B2 (see them under these headings).

Nutrient The food substances necessary for growth and health. Examples of nutrients are protein, carbohydrates, and water.

Obesity The condition of being extremely overweight.

Omega-3 Fatty acids from seafood. Unlike most fats, omega-3 has a type of cholesterol that seems to help prevent heart disease.

Osteoporosis A weak-bone disease usually occurring later in life. More common in females, osteoporosis is believed to be the result of a diet low in calcium (the mineral found in dairy products, fish, dark green vegetables, and almonds) and too little exercise (see "Exercise").

Pita bread A Mediterranean bread made from a fibrous plant flour, shaped like a pouch which forms a pocket inside.

Poach To simmer food that's soaked in a liquid. The liquid may be water, or wine but not oil or butter, in which case it would be sautéing.

Polyunsaturated fat Fat found mostly in specific plant foods, such as vegetable oil, corn oil, and margarine.

GLOSSARY

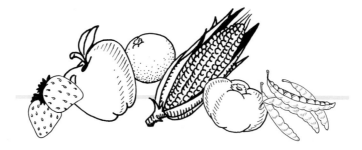

Potassium A mineral that helps muscles and the heart function properly. Some good sources of potassium are bananas, oranges, and dried fruits.

Preservatives Chemicals added to foods to prevent spoilage or the growth of harmful bacteria. Some preservatives are salt, sugar, ethyl formate, and sorbic acid.

"Prime" meat A United States Department of Agriculture label identifying the meat with the most fat, compared to "choice," "good," "lean," and "extra lean." Prime meat is also more expensive.

Processed See Refined.

Protein A nutrient that builds and repairs body tissue, fights infection, and provides energy. Sources of protein are meat, dried beans, poultry, dairy products, egg whites, and nuts.

Puberty The period from age 9 to 18 when children develop into adults (see "Sex & Hormonal Changes").

Recommended Daily Allowances (RDA) The United States government's estimate of a healthy person's daily nutritional needs, which includes carbohydrates, fat, fiber, protein, vitamins, and minerals. Do not worry about getting *all* of these nutrients, but aim for them.

"Reduced calorie" A Food & Drug Administration label identifying a product with one-third fewer calories than it would normally have.

Refined A machine or chemical process that changes food from its most natural state.

Riboflavin See Vitamin B2.

Ricotta A white Italian cheese that resembles cottage cheese.

Roast To cook (usually meat) uncovered in an oven or over an open fire or charcoal.

Saccharin A low-calorie artificial sweetener.

Safflower oil Liquid fat made from a thistle-like herb. It can be used in salad, margarine, and other foods.

Salivary glands Tissues in the cheeks that secrete saliva ("spit") to help "water down" the food in your mouth for swallowing.

Salt (sodium chloride) A food substance found in trace amounts from foods in their natural state. Large amounts of sodium are also added to canned soups, canned vegetables, pickles, ketchup, dry cereal, and other packaged foods. Sodium has been found to complicate high blood pressure, which can lead to heart disease.

GLOSSARY

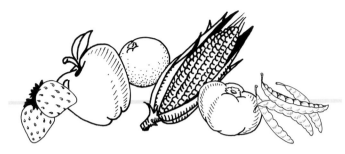

Saturated fat Problem fat usually found in meat and dairy products (bacon, meat, butter, cheese) and some vegetable products (palm oil, palm kernel oil and coconut oil). Saturated fat tends to increase cholesterol levels in the blood.

Sauté To cook food rapidly in an open pan with a small amount of fat or oil.

Scurvy A disease caused by lack of vitamin C in the diet. Symptoms include slow-healing wounds, shortness of breath, swollen and bleeding gums, and the loosening or loss of teeth.

Simple carbohydrates (sugar) The sweet-tasting substance found naturally in some foods, such as milk and fruit. Visible sugars such as white and brown, have been changed from natural sugars.

Skim milk Milk from which as much fat as possible has been removed, compared to low-fat milk, which has some fat removed, and whole milk, which has the highest fat content.

Small intestine See Intestines.

Sodium chloride See Salt.

Soft cheeses Muenster, limburger, blue, Brie, Camembert, ricotta, cottage, Gorgonzola, Roquefort, Stilton, brick, Port du Salut, Trappist, Wensleydale, Bel Paese, Neufchatel, bakers', cream, pot, primost, and myost.

Sorbitol A natural sweetener found in berries, cherries, plums, pears, apples, and blackstrap molasses. It is used in many manufactured foods, including chewing gum, dry roasted nuts, icing, and shredded coconut.

Sparkling water Bottled water that contains bubbles made by carbon dioxide gas.

Starch See Complex Carbohydrates

Steam To cook food by exposing it to the vapor from a boiling liquid.

Stew To cook food in a seasoned liquid for a long time at low temperatures.

Stimulant A substance that increases the body's awareness or ability to function in different ways. Caffeine from tablets or coffee are examples of stimulants (see "Substance Abuse").

Stir-fry To cook food quickly in a little fat or oil by constantly moving it in a hot skillet or wok.

Stress The strain a person experiences under certain physical (illness, injury, environment) or mental conditions (fear, anger, anxiety) (see "Stress & Mental Health").

Sugar (1) Sweet crystals from sugarcane or sugar beet plants (sucrose); (2) Foods containing an excessive amount of sugar (see also Carbohydrates, Simple); (3) A number of sweet

GLOSSARY

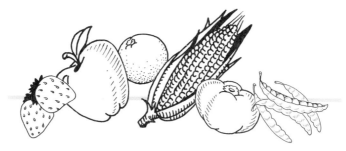

substances, such as fructose and dextrose, made partly from natural sources and added to foods.

Supplement A preparation of minerals or vitamins, usually in tablet form, used to provide additional nutrients to the diet.

Thiamine See Vitamin B1.

Tofu A white, nearly tasteless blend of soybeans and water from Asia. It usually comes in a dense, congealed square and is smooth and slightly chewy. Not only is it very low in calories, but it is cholesterol-free and high in many nutrients.

Urination Passing liquid waste and excess out of the body.

Veal Meat from a cow slaughtered at a young age. Visually, veal is leaner than regular beef, but also more expensive.

Vegetarian A person who eats a diet consisting of only vegetables.

Vegetarian diet A diet that consists only of plant foods; no meat, fish, or other animal products are included.

Vitamin Food elements needed by the body for normal growth and function.

Vitamin A An element necessary for growth, healthy eyes, skin, and linings of the throat and digestive tract. Some good sources of Vitamin A are eggs, low-fat cheese and dark green, yellow, and orange fruits and vegetables.

Vitamin B1 or Thiamine An element necessary for the nervous system. Vitamin B1 also helps the body turn food into energy. Some good sources of Vitamin B1 are ham, oysters, whole-grain and enriched cereals, pastas and bread, peas, and lima beans.

Vitamin B2 or Riboflavin An element that helps the body use oxygen. Vitamin B2 is also good for the skin. Some good sources of Vitamin B2 are skim milk, low-fat meat, whole-grain and enriched breads, dark green vegetables, mushrooms, and dried beans.

Vitamin B6 An element that helps the body absorb protein. Some good sources of Vitamin B6 are whole-grain (but not enriched) cereals and breads, spinach, green beans, fish, and poultry.

Vitamin B12 An element that helps the body use protein, fat, and carbohydrates. Vitamin B12 also helps the body produce red blood cells. Some good sources of Vitamin B12 are found only in animal foods such as low-fat meat and milk, fish, and oysters.

GLOSSARY

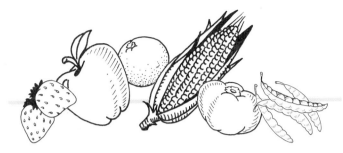

Vitamin C An element that helps keep gums healthy and hold body cells together. Some good sources of Vitamin C are citrus fruits, and dark green vegetables.

Vitamin D An element that helps the body absorb calcium for strong bones and teeth. Some good sources of Vitamin D are low-fat milk and other dairy products, salmon, and eggs.

Vitamin E An element that helps the body produce red blood cells, muscles, and other tissues. Vitamin E also helps protect vitamin A. Some good sources of Vitamin E are vegetable oils, whole-grain cereals and breads; dried beans, and green, leafy vegetables.

Water The most important nutrient for life, water composes 50 to 60 percent of our bodies.

Whole grain A plant food in which the kernel is whole. None of the three parts of the kernel have been removed, like they have in white flour, white rice, and wheat bread. Examples of whole-grain foods are bran cereal, cornbread, oatmeal, whole-wheat flour, and brown rice.

Whole milk Milk with the most amount of fat, compared to skim milk and low-fat milk.

Xylitol A sweetener that can be made from berries, leaves, mushrooms, or chemicals. It is used in manufactured products like dietary foods and chewing gum.

Yo-yo syndrome The act of continually gaining, then losing, then gaining weight over again.

Zinc A mineral that aids appetite and growth. Some sources of zinc are low-fat meat, eggs, and seafood.

27386

613   Spence, Annette c.2
S   Nutrition

$18.95

DATE			